John, Dementia

by

Rosemary Westwell

To Dr. Dening
with many thanks
Rosemary Westwell 27/01/2013

Copyright Rosemary Westwell 2012

North Staffordshire Press Ltd
Stoke-on-Trent
Staffordshire

John, Dementia and Me

All Rights Reserved

ISBN 978-0-9574416-0-6

First Published in 2012
By
North Staffordshire Press
Staffordshire University Business Village
72 Leek Road, Stoke-on-Trent, Staffordshire
United Kingdom

Printed and bound by Design Bindings Ltd, Staffordshire
Cover design by Lee Holland Illustration

Acknowledgements

Grateful thanks to Alzheimer's Research UK and everyone who helped in the production of this book. Special thanks to Dr Dening for his invaluable support during our experiences as described in the novel and for his excellent foreword, to Mary McGuire for the title, and all the family and friends who have patiently assisted me through my experiences and in the making of this book.

Foreword

Dementia is perhaps the ultimate human challenge. Our powers of thinking, of language, and all the ways in which we relate to the world and communicate with each other are what separate us from other species and make us into the human beings that we are. Dementia erodes our mental powers and in doing so asks important questions about life and personhood. We fear it as an irreversible medical condition yet we also have much to learn from it, both about the brain and how it works but also about the people that we are now and may become in the future.

The term dementia applies to a state of having irreversible cognitive impairment severe enough to interfere with everyday living. So it is more than just getting slightly forgetful as we get older, though it can be difficult to distinguish where forgetfulness ends and dementia starts to take over, especially at the outset. The commonest cause of dementia is Alzheimer's disease, which is so common that the term is used almost interchangeably with dementia itself. However, other brain diseases can also produce dementia, and these may cause different characteristic changes in mental functioning and behaviour as they progress.

One important form of dementia that is separate from Alzheimer's disease is known as frontotemporal dementia because of the areas of the brain most typically affected. It is probably a group of diseases as we know that in some cases there is an inherited genetic basis and in other cases this is less clear. The term Pick's disease is sometimes used though this more accurately applies to people with certain types of microscopic changes in their brains, not something we can see during their lives however. People with frontotemporal dementia may present with speech problems – difficulty finding words or else not speaking at all – but if the frontal lobes are mainly affected the characteristic changes are in behaviour. Sometimes, people with this condition start to behave in bizarre, disinhibited ways that can be embarrassing or even dangerous, for example in relation to driving or using machinery. This condition often presents at a younger age than Alzheimer's dementia so the effects of a middle aged person, perhaps at the height of their career and with a young family at home, developing this disorder can be absolutely devastating.

Rosemary Westwell has walked this journey alongside someone with frontotemporal dementia. In this book, she charts the changes in his behaviour, the unpredictability of life with dementia, and how hard it can be to know how to respond. One of the interesting threads is how some of the behaviour was there all along and it was the intensity and frequency of oddness that increased. From my own experience of patients with frontotemporal dementia, there is often a long trace into the past that suggests the dementia has a developmental as well as a degenerative aspect. Rosemary has let the events within the home tell the story so the doctors and other services take a back seat, an important reminder to us professionals that we only see a fraction of what goes on. And at the end, is John there or not? The reader can decide for themselves.

Dr Tom Dening
Consultant Psychiatrist & Medical Director, Cambridgeshire & Peterborough NHS Foundation Trust.

Chapter 1

I pressed the container hard and caught the squirt of alcohol. Rubbing my hands together again and again, I prepared myself for the ordeal. I needed time — time to summon up enough courage not to leave.

There was a movement in the corridor ahead. I turned my eyes away from the noise. If I saw what was happening through the glass in the door, I might use it as an excuse not to go in. No, I was going in no matter what. I began to tap the numbers into the keypad. Before completing the code, I could not contain myself any longer. I glanced into the corridor.

A tall thin man, wild eyes flickering, rushed towards me. He pressed his nose hard against the window, his face looking like a battered boxer. Drat! He was there again. I should have felt sorry for the chap, his failing mind forcing him to live in an alien and unfriendly world, but I didn't. I didn't feel sorry for him, I felt annoyed that he was there and that I would have to battle my way past him to get to see my husband, whom I did not especially want to see either. I rubbed my left wrist. The bruises were still fresh from last time. I hated it when the patients grabbed me. I knew they only wanted a bit of human contact. They were not trying to molest me, but I felt molested, soiled, as if what they had was catching and if I didn't get away from them soon I would end up like them. Thank goodness for Babs. At least this time I was armed with a little knowledge that might help. Babs and I had been having our weekly

1

morning coffee together. She had her head cocked to one side, listening patiently to me going on and on about how I hated visiting John because the inmates grabbed me so that I couldn't get away.

'You can holler as much as you like for a care assistant or a nurse,' I moaned, 'but they're always busy doing something else, like taking an inmate to the toilet.'

'I can show you one thing, if you like.' Babs shook her mass of curls so that they partly masked the smile that she was trying to hide. She was always so competent, nothing worried her. She sailed through life as though it were permanently problem free. She had no idea.

'Please do!' I snapped, slightly annoyed that she found my predicament amusing.

'Well, if a patient grabs you by the wrist ...'

'Which they often do,' I interjected.'

'Simply turn your hand towards their thumb and you will be able to release your hand.'

'Oh yeah,' I sneered, not ready to be eased out of my bad mood so quickly.

'Here, try.' Babs grabbed my hand.

'Let go!' I shrieked involuntarily. Oh how I hated my hand being grabbed. Babs clung on. With a disgruntled sigh, I stared at her hand firmly wrapped around my wrist. She still had a tan from her holiday abroad. Her grip was so tight.

'Go on, try it,' she urged me again.

'Oh, all right then.' I could see that I had at least to pretend to struggle before she would let go. I looked at her thumb.

'Turn my hand towards your thumb, you said.'

'That's right.'

I wished her eyes would stop twinkling. She was enjoying this. Slowly I turned my hand towards her wrist. She held on firmly, but the more I turned my hand and pushed hard towards her thumb, the weaker her grip became. Suddenly I wrenched my hand free.

'I did it!' I shrieked. 'By Jove, I did it! Oh, thank you, Babs!' I hugged her with almost as much force as she had gripped my hand.

'It's OK,' Babs mumbled, still smothered in my hug. 'You can let go of me now.' She took in a large gulp of air after I finally released her.

The care home door rattled. The wild-eyed man was still there.

'I want to go out!' His muffled voice sounded urgent. Well, he can't go out. The care assistants have enough problems without having to chase him around the home if I let him out. Behind the grinning face, the long grey carpet was empty. He was now moving restlessly from side to side. There were no members of staff. Well, I couldn't stand here all day. I had to go in some time. My heart thumped.

I planned my manoeuvres. I would finish tapping in the code and quickly grab the door handle ready for a tug of war with the man. With my left hand gripping the door handle hard, I would turn my right shoulder towards the opening in the doorway and fight my way in by pushing him back further inside with my shoulder. At least, that was the plan.

'Oh, there you are, George.' A plump woman rushed down the corridor, her rolls of fat bouncing as she advanced. She stood next to the wild-eyed inmate.

'Come on now, let the lady through. You have to come with me to the sitting room.' The care assistant took the man's arm gently, giving me a placatory smile. He resisted for a moment. The care assistant's strong authoritative voice spoke again.

'Now come on, George. You know you shouldn't stand here.' Reluctantly, the patient let the care assistant lead him away.

Hands shaking, I finished punching the numbers into the keypad and the door clicked open. I pulled it back, rushed through and closed it behind me quickly, just in case.

Room number 27 was on my left. The photo of my husband beside the door peered up at me. His head was at an awkward angle. It was obvious the disease had taken its effect. His eyes in the photo were dull and confused. I glanced up and down the corridor. There was no sign of George or the care assistant. I knocked on the door. There was no reply. I opened it and saw a shape in the hospital bed. Classical music was playing quietly from a radio on the table in the corner.

His head turned quickly in my direction. His pale blue eyes were wide, the whites bright and unfriendly.

'Hello, John,' I said, trying to sound cheerful.
He stared.

'So, how are you today? Do you recognize me?'
His eyes remained fixed. They did not change. He held the side of the bed firmly, his body twisted and immobile.

'Well, I don't know,' I continued, 'married to you for nigh on 30 years and you don't even recognize me!'

A light glimmered in his eyes. He grinned. He did recognize me!

He made a sound. It was the sound of recognition a baby gives before it has learnt to speak but it was a man's deep voice.

'Can you say my name?' I wondered why I was asking him to do this. What purpose was there in asking him to try to do something that he was no longer capable of doing? His lips moved into an awkward shape.

'Al,' he said. 'Al,' he tried again. He was nearly there, although to others my name would be unrecognizable.

'Yes, that's right. It's your wife, Sally, who has come to visit you.'

He looked at me fixedly. Sadly I returned his fixed gaze. Why was I there? What could I do? I could not have any kind of conversation with my husband any more. I could talk to him, but he could not respond. Besides, did he understand what I said? Did he understand anything at all?

I wanted to turn around and go straight out of the room. I wanted to leave there and then. He would not know or care, would he? Why did I torment us both by coming every month to try to rekindle what was once between us?

Feelings of resentment clouded my thinking. I married John for this? He was nothing like the man I had married so many years ago. His promises of a joyful life together had been destroyed. I looked at my husband. He was a shell of a man, trapped in a deformed body. Why was he being kept alive like this? You would not wish this on your worst enemy. Sinister thoughts continued to stir in my mind. I would deal with them later. The body before me, the remaining fragments of the handsome young man I had married, was now a man who could not move, who was in nappies, who could not speak, and who could not feed himself. This was not my John.

I stopped. But it was my John. He was still there behind those suffering eyes that could still smile. He tried to speak again, his grunts a little longer this time. His noises said to me that he was there. He was still alive and still wanted to see me at his bedside. He still wanted to claim me as his soul mate, his woman.

'You knew you'd got a bargain when you married me, didn't you?' I said. His smile did not alter.

Suddenly my spine chilled. I felt a presence immediately behind me. Someone had crept into the room and was breathing heavily down my neck.

'Have you got a car?' The man's voice was urgent, aggressive and right in my left ear. I turned to face the drugged eyes of a slight figure, padding from one foot to the other. Now what should I do?

'Have you got a car?' his hand suddenly reached for mine and he gripped hard. Oh, not again.

'Nurse?' I craned my neck to look behind him. There was no response. My heart hammered. Quick! What did Babs say? Turn your hand towards his thumb.

'Sorry, mate.' Angrily I forced my hand over towards his thumb. 'I don't have a car!' I tried not to shriek with the annoyance and fear I felt. I released my hand suddenly. I moved quickly to the door. How was I going to get him out of here? The figure had hardly noticed the way I had wrenched my hand away from him. He touched John's bedside table and, swaying gently, loomed over the body of John. What if he molested John? How could I stop him? As with John, his illness probably made him strong, stronger than he would have been before he became ill. I stepped outside into the corridor frantically looking for staff. The corridor was still empty. My heart thumping loudly in my chest, I gripped the door handle and glared at the patient, willing him to leave. He turned around. How could I be frightened of this beaten man, his shabby clothes, his hunched shoulders and uncertain movements? Then his eyes made contact. The whites stood out starkly in the shadow. He dithered. I gulped and hurriedly stepped back, hiding my free hand. He slowly padded forward and out into the corridor busy in his own world of confusion. I leaned right back as he walked directly in front of me. He smelt of urine. Finally he was outside the door. I let out a sigh of relief. I quickly closed the door, pulled the chair closer to John's bed and sat down.

The room was quiet save for the gentle classical music playing — Mozart's 40th symphony. That strange melancholic but energetic opening fitted my mood exactly. John's head was resting on his chest, his hand still clutching the side of his bed. He was absent from the world for the moment. I tried to ignore the sickly sweet whiff of nappies as I put my hand gently onto his. He lifted his head and looked directly at me but his expression was dull.

'Do you remember when we first met?' He yawned, revealing a row of ruined teeth. 'I had come over from Australia. You had just come back from a trip to Toronto in the summer of 1973.'

I looked outside the window. The sky was a clear pale blue, much paler than the sky when I first left Tasmania.

Chapter 2

I was 24. The sunlit town of Devonport, Tasmania, Australia, faded away as the plane flew over my house and the houses of my various discarded boyfriends. Was I doing the right thing? Should I have stayed with my dad in that large, rambling house? No, there was no going back. I had to believe what I was doing was right.

I was leaving behind the world of political manoeuvrings and the intransigent Education Department. My heart was cold, the same coldness I had felt when I had left school and university. Why cry about change that was inevitable? It was no good dwelling on the past. I was not sorry to turn my back on being bullied at boarding school. I was not sorry to leave behind the people who had taught me that love was a passion that had to be kept under lock and key and that the more you let yourself be overwhelmed by your feelings for someone you thought special, the greater the heartbreak when you realized that you were not the only soul mate of someone you adored. No, I was not sorry to put all of this behind me. I would not allow my heart to be broken again. I would be in control from now on.

John stirred in his bed in the care home.

'Do you remember that night at the Young Conservative do? You took my friend Dave off to play mini golf, leaving me high and dry, didn't you?'

The sky outside his window was now filled with billowing clouds. John stared blankly.

'But I didn't let you forget it, did I?'

The pub where the Young Conservatives were meeting was full. Dave Fennel and I were just friends, no more. In our early twenties we had the world to conquer. We had plenty of time. Dave stood at the bar, tall and thin, a likeable young man, as casual a member of the Young Conservatives as I was. We were just finishing a quiet drink before joining the others for a session of mini golf when a short moustached stranger clapped Dave's shoulder.

'Hello there, Dave, how are you? At the watering hole already, I see. Would you like me to buy you a drink?'

'No, I'm all right, thanks.' Dave put his drink down and shook the stranger's hand. 'I haven't seen you for ages! Where have you been?'

'I've just returned from Toronto — last night, in fact. Fantastic city. You've never seen such tall buildings. Are you ready for a game of mini golf? Come on then.'

Dave downed the remainder of his drink and they turned their backs and walked away.

Open-mouthed I stood alone at the bar. How dare this interloper intervene! It was not only his intervention that annoyed me, it was the fact that I had made no impression on him whatsoever. How dare he *ignore me*! I couldn't really blame Dave, we were just having a casual drink, and we had not officially decided we would be playing a game of mini golf together, it had been assumed. However, the interloper should have seen that we were having a drink together and that maybe *he* was the gooseberry, the third person, the one *we* should have asked if *he* wanted to join *us*, not the other way round. Even then, *I* had been completely ignored. No, I was not going to let this go. I was not going to be snubbed by such a short, smooth-talking smart — I decided not to try any more to find the right word to express exactly what I thought of him. Whatever he was, I would have my revenge.

'So, you had a good game with my friend Dave?' I tried to curb the acidity of my tone as I stood in front of this short, young man, his moustache and his smoothed short-cropped hair perfectly in place.

'Yes,' he grinned showing a row of perfectly white teeth. 'He won but as Churchill says: "Golf is a game whose aim is to hit a very small ball into an even smaller hole, with weapons singularly ill-designed for the purpose."'

The corners of my mouth twitched but I would not give in to a smile, not yet.

'You know you went off with my friend, Dave. He and I were getting ready to play a game together and you butted in.'

'Did I?' his rich voice underlined his reply with such sincerity I almost believed him. 'I'm *so* sorry.' He was a real charmer; there was no doubt about that. I watched him closely as he glanced towards the crush of people at the bar.

'Can I get you a drink?' he asked, using that same tone of sincerity and concern. I was still not certain whether it was all charm or whether he meant it. Best to play it safe.

'Yeah,' I drawled, my Aussie accent still strongly in place. 'I'll have a brandy and dry, please.'

'Brandy and dry. Dry, what do you mean by dry?' he looked at me for the first time.

'You Poms don't know what 'dry' means?' I laughed, overdoing the indignity for his benefit. His grin broadened. 'It's dry ginger ale.'

'Oh, right. Brandy and dry it is then.'

There was no getting away from it — like Napoleon, he was short, but he was very smartly dressed and he bore what height he had with an air of unquestionable authority. His voice had an appealing depth and potency. I could listen to him for hours.

He chatted excitedly with the others at the bar while he waited for our drinks.

'Thank you,' I said as he put my brandy and dry down on the table in front of me and sat on the stool opposite.

'My name is John by the way.' He put his drink down and offered his hand. I half stood up and shook it. His grip was firm and confident.

'Sally,' I said and sat down. 'How long have you been a member of the Young Conservatives?' I asked taking a sip of the brandy and dry. Oh how I wished the Poms would keep their dry ginger in the fridge. Were all their drinks warm like this?

'For a while.' He was now looking at me, probably weighing me up. Did he approve or not? I could not be sure. Why did it matter, anyway? His eyes were a very pale blue and yet his hair was light brown, not blond.

'After I left the Coffee Pot Club, I decided to join the Young Conservatives. It is very important that we win the next election.'

Uh-oh. He was a political fanatic. Still, I had decided that politics here would be different from the politics in Tassie and I had had enough of them. At least this country was much larger and more important. I quickly changed the subject.

'What was the Coffee Pot Club?'

'Oh, it was just a group of us who wanted to socialize. I met my ex-fiancée there.'

Ex-fiancée? So he's interested in the idea of marriage. What was she like? What stopped them getting married? I should have read the warning signs but before I could start this line of questioning, John was steaming ahead.

'We're meeting at the Green Man again next Saturday. I think I'll go.' He sipped his beer. 'What do you do?'

His blue eyes looked into mine. Why didn't he ask if I would come with him to the Green Man? Really, this chap was impossible.

'I'm a teacher. I teach at a comprehensive school in Peterborough. It's jolly hard work and by the weekend I'm really ready for a break, but I find the weekends so boring.' This should do the trick.

'Yes, they can be, can't they? I take my mother out sometimes. It keeps her sweet.'

Great! This was definitely a bit of a dead duck. No budding romance likely to bloom here. At least he was taking his mother out and not another girlfriend.

'Well, must go.' I finished the last of my brandy and dry. If he were not going to ask me out, I could at least make my mark on him by leaving early.

He raised his eyebrows. 'Must you?'

''Fraid so, piles of books to mark,' I lied. 'I'm staying with a lovely old lady, Mrs Edwards, at Manor Farm in Eastborough, if you ever want to get in contact with me again. It's in the phone book.'

'How are you getting home?' he stood up. 'I could give you a lift if you liked.'

'Thank you, but I have my own car. I'll see you around, eh?'

I made a beeline for the door. He stood very still, watching my early exit. 'Keep 'em wanting more.' I muttered to myself.

The body in front of me coughed, wracked in a paroxysm of pain. Was John in pain or was he just coughing loudly because he can? He no longer behaved as the gentleman I first knew. Now he was completely uninhibited. He had no understanding of how he should behave. He could do and say and act in any way he liked. I patted his hand.

'It was Mrs Edwards' grandson who answered your phone call, wasn't it?'

John's cold eyes stared. There was still no recognition.

'Trust my luck to be out when you called. Fortunately Victor left a message that you had phoned otherwise we would never have met again. Do you remember Mrs Edwards and her lovely old house?'

A cloud moved slowly across the pale blue sky outside. I sighed.

I could see Mrs Edwards now, a darling little dumpling of an old lady living in the Manor, Eastborough. It was a large brick house nestled amongst the trees at the entrance to an extensive farm. I fell in love with the house the moment I saw it. Stepping into the dark interior, onto the old misshapen flagstones, I could feel the laughter and warmth of the many, busy inhabitants who had been born, had loved, had worked and probably had died there. Even though the dear old lady was the only occupant, I felt the house wrap itself around me, hugging me, making me feel more welcome than I had ever felt in the three years I had been in the country.

My husband turned his head away from me suddenly. Something on the wall next to him fascinated him. The wall was blank. Was there any point in my continuing? I stood up to go. His head turned back. His eyes pleaded with me. In a split second, he was there with me. He did not want me to go. Didn't he always do that? Every time I decided to do something, such as when I was preparing to go out to an important event, just as I was about to open the door, or when I was waiting for a phone call and it finally rang, he always managed to stop me by doing something drastic like knocking a hole in a water pipe, crashing his head into a wall, or dropping something fragile so that it smashed to pieces.

The room in the care home was quiet except for the classical music and the shuffle of feet outside the door. The feet stopped. I took in a sharp breath and stood up ready for another incident — not again, please not again. The feet then moved on. I sat down on the chair and sighed.

'You finally invited me out and took me to the Green Man, didn't you?'

Chapter 3

The pub was set amongst leafy trees in a village in the country. It was a small pub with thick, newly laid thatch hanging over its tiny windows. We walked in. The pub interior was dark; old wooden beams and brasses surrounded the bar; the atmosphere was busy, friendly and inviting. It was a long way from the spit and sawdust pubs I had seen in Tasmania. Here, it was grace and charm; in Tasmania, a girl was hardly allowed to set foot inside a pub.

'I'll have a double brandy and dry this time, please.' John's mouth dropped open. He closed it quickly and, without a word, went to buy the drinks.

'So, what do you do as a job?' I asked him as he set the drinks down.

'I work for Nelson and Hall, selling pesticides and herbicides.' His smart suit, pristine shirt and conservative tie certainly looked the part. If I were a farmer I would certainly have bought from him, but it was too soon to admit the attraction.

'So you are one of these terrible people who are poisoning the countryside, eh?'

'Something like that,' he grinned, 'but that's as may be. You know we have increased food production incredibly with these new products. There are far too many people for our land to be able to feed them without the help we give.'

I sipped my drink quietly as he enthused over his job, his life, his company car and the friends he had made.

'I have a lot of farming friends. Maybe you'd like to come with me on one of my rounds?'

At last, an invitation, but when? 'That would be great,' I said. To meet real farming folk, as a friend of a local inhabitant would be so much better than the cold and distant introductions I had had so far. But I did not pin my hopes on his carrying out his promise. I downed the drink and asked for another.

The body next to me moved his hand away, his head bowed. His fingers pulled at the blankets covering him in a rhythmic gesture that meant something only to him, if it meant anything at all. There were agitated voices in the corridor. I listened, but they did not come any closer to John's room.

'It was on the second date that you told me all about your mother, wasn't it?' I tried hard to keep the bitterness out of my tone.

After our second round of drinks, after the jokes and witticisms, John let me see a tiny glimpse of the shadows in his life, shadows that were to haunt our marriage for all time.

'When my dad died, it was so unexpected. If it wasn't for me, he might be alive today.' He looked down at the table.

'No, that can't be true!' I said, the sympathetic tone in my voice stronger than I intended.

He looked up at me briefly. 'My mother is finding it very difficult to cope. I do the best I can to keep her happy.' He frowned. 'She's always been difficult, especially since Dad died. Nothing seems to please her.' My maternal instincts stirred. Poor lad. He has had a hard time of it. He looked into his glass.

'Dad died the day after I left home to move into a flat on my own.'

I paused, stopping myself from blurting out 'So what?'

'You mustn't feel guilty about your father,' I said steadying my voice, carefully. 'Most children think they're responsible for a parent's death when it happens, but it's simply not true. People die and there is no escape from it.' I put my hand on his.

He continued to stare at his drink 'But mother —'

'No, you mustn't think that your moving out could possibly have killed your father. Do you mind if I ask what he died of?'

'Well, after some trouble with his brother he became run down and he got the flu, which developed into pneumonia.'

'Exactly,' I said. 'What was the trouble with his brother?'

John frowned. 'I'd rather not go into that now, if you don't mind.'

I searched for his gaze. 'For me it was my mum, who died of cancer when she was young — only 49. It took me a good five years to get over it.' I sipped the brandy and dry. 'Actually, you never get over it do you?' I looked hard at his troubled face, willing him to look at me.

John paused and looked down. 'I had a terrible nightmare when Dad died. I imagined an atomic bomb had gone off. It was frightening.' He released his hand and gripped his pint firmly. 'I've never told anyone this before.' He paused again for a moment and then looked up suddenly. 'Would you like to come away with me for the weekend?'

My mouth gaped. I quickly brought my lips together and checked his expression. Did he really ask me away for the weekend, so soon?

He looked at me earnestly. 'I'm going to stay with very close friends of mine who run a farm in Essex. Would you like to come with me?'

The weekend? His shoulders were square, his features inscrutable. He really meant it. We barely knew each other. We had been going out for a total of three weeks. I glanced at him again. He didn't look like the last cad who had asked me away for the weekend. The last time I went away I had trusted my friend completely, only to discover that at the party we attended he found a lost love and he remained glued to her for the rest of the evening. I spent the night listening to their love making in the room above. Great! I would never let something like *that* happen again. In future, I determined, I would have enough money for a taxi home!

John looked at me, grinning, expectant.

'Yes, I'd love to.' I tried to sound convinced.

'Do you remember that weekend?' A flicker of recognition sparked in John's eyes as he turned to smile at me. The room in the care home seemed to light up with new warmth.

'You wanted to go for a walk, and I couldn't be bothered?' His face was suddenly dull again. It was as though he had suddenly turned into a perfect stranger, his blank expression lacking all emotion. I stared out of the window, pretending I was not affected by the change.

The summer of 1973 was a good one. On the day John and I set off for our weekend away, the sun was shining strongly and the summer sky was pale and clear as I climbed into his Ford Escort, my purse bulging with enough money for a taxi ride home. I was very comfortable, sitting in the passenger seat next to this young, confident new friend. There was something special about having a man take you away in his car for a weekend. I could get used to this life.

'We will be staying with my best friends, Bill and Mary,' John said. We were speeding along the A10, fields hidden by rows of trees, the road full of cars — far more than I was used to seeing in Tasmania. He changed gear and then slowed to go round a roundabout. He turned the wheel and, with years of practice, negotiated the exit without a hitch. 'I've known them for years. They have a pig farm.'

A pig farm? Aren't they smelly places to avoid? I grimaced. But a farm is a farm, and pigs or not, I was looking forward to going to stay on a real farm in England. Fields of golden wheat and barley stretched on either side of the road as we sped towards Great Dunmow. The flat lands of the Fens had begun to undulate.

'Hills, real hills. It's ages since I've seen some hills,' I joked. John grinned and concentrated on his driving. Closer to our destination, the roads became very narrow and were lined by high hedges. There must be a lot of accidents on these roads, I thought. How were people to know if someone were speeding round the corner straight into your path? You certainly couldn't see them.

John gave a loud blast on the horn. 'That's to let anyone around the corner know we're coming.' It was as though he had read my thoughts. 'I haven't been here for a while, but I'm quite sure I know the way,' he continued. The village sign said Broxted.

I was happy to travel for some distance yet. The scenery was so beautiful — picture box tableaux of the English countryside. Small thatched cottages painted light pink were gathered together into quaint little pockets as we sped from one village to another.

'Oh.' John pulled up onto the grass verge. The sign in front of us said Broxted, again. 'I think I must have taken a wrong turning.'

I folded my arms. John put the car into reverse, backed and turned to face a different direction and we sped off again. We saw the sign for Broxted two more times. Was this assured individual as competent as he looked? Could I believe anything he said? In fact, could he be trusted at all? I clutched my handbag firmly, reassured that the taxi money was still there.

'Ah, *this* is the way.' He turned into a road I had not seen before. The roads narrowed again and we finally pulled up at a large thatched cottage that looked directly onto an unsealed lane. Ancient trees lined the road and the fields beyond were bursting, ready for harvesting.

As John put on the handbrake two smiling people emerged from the cottage.

'Welcome!' said a smooth-faced woman, hugging John. A slim, tanned man stood close behind her. John came round to my side to open the door.

'This is Sally. Sally, meet Mary and Bill.' John's voice was tinged with pride.

I clambered out of the car and shook their hands. Their handshakes were warm and welcoming.

'Pleased to meet you.' I bowed my head in a sudden attack of shyness.

'Come in, come in.' Mary led the way and John shepherded me behind them into the cool dark cottage.

'Do sit down. Would you like some tea?' Mary spoke from the kitchen, a tray already set, the kettle boiling on the fuel stove.

I chose an armchair that did not look as if it had been occupied for a while. I sat on the edge.

'How's the farm?' John asked Bill.

'It's been a difficult year. The pig market is not good.' As the two friends talked farming, I looked around the room. It was comfortable, with a lived-in look, but tidy and clean. The shelves were filled with books, the kind of books I liked — factual: about birds, plants, art; and a good dose of crime fiction, with a full row of Agatha Christie. I was itching to get at them but I looked at the two friends talking earnestly about their business. I did not want to disturb them.

Tea arrived.

'Milk and sugar?' Mary asked me.

'Just milk, please.'

She poured a little milk into a blue china cup, put a tea strainer over it and poured the tea. Her movements were calm, experienced.

'Would you like a piece of cake?'

'Yes, please.' The cake was a large Madeira, with a number of red cherries on top. The teacup rattled as I balanced it on my lap reaching forward to accept a rather large piece of the cake. I'll diet after the weekend, I thought.

'Have you got a lot for us to do this weekend?' John leaned forward, his tea and cake left on the arm of his chair as an afterthought.

'We've a couple of fields to harvest. We should be able to do it over the weekend.' Bill sat back in his chair and cut his slice of cake with the edge of his fork and ate it.

'So, how's your mother, John?' Mary brought her own tea and cake to sit near us.

John's shoulders stiffened. 'Oh, she's not so bad. I took her shopping yesterday. She really needs someone to help her. You can choose your friends, but you can't choose your relatives, eh?' He grinned, his eyes unable to hide a residue of concern.

Mary patted his hand, 'She'll come round. You must be strong and not let her interfere with your friendships. You know I saw her sisters in Cambridge last week. The Cox family certainly know how to keep their looks, don't they?'

'Yes, I suppose so,' sighed John. Then, changing the subject, he asked brightly, 'Where are the boys?'

'They're away for the weekend. It's a pity you've missed them. More tea?' Mary smiled at me. I could not resist. It had a unique taste. It was not the usual British tea I had been having.

Mary topped up my teacup and asked, 'Have you helped with a harvest before?'

'No, this is my first time. I'm looking forward to it.'

'I hope you have brought some sturdy clothes and shoes. It can be quite rough work sometimes. Let me know if you want anything. I'm sure I could find something if you need it.'

'That's kind. Thank you.' I pulled my skirt down; making sure it covered my knees.

'When we've finished I will show you to your separate rooms.' I wasn't sure but I thought the word 'separate' was emphasized just a little more than necessary. I wondered if Bill and Mary had been having some discussion about the bedding arrangements.

'No more?' Mary took my cup and saucer, put them on the tray and took them to the kitchen.

I stood up. 'Can I help with the washing up?'

'No, it's all right. I'll deal with it in a minute. Let me show you to your room. John, you have David's room, All right?'

I followed Mary up the stairs. They were narrow and dark; the walls were thick, wooden and black. It was like stepping back into a timeless age. It was as though nothing had changed from the days when people farmed without machines, or technology, when they had fed themselves from the harvest they had collected with sheer physical hard work.

'Watch your head!' Mary said just before I entered the doorway into the front room that was to be mine. The door latch was a simple affair, like the one on our lavatory in the back shed at home.

Chapter 4

I awoke the next morning, in the country farmhouse, to the sound of birdsong. Even the birdsong was gentler and more charming than the raucous calls I used to hear at home in Tasmania. The sun shone in streams of warm sharp beams that spread over the counterpane. This was bliss. I could see the lush green trees across the lane through the tiny square windowpanes.

John and I sat close at the breakfast table. The sun was shining through the leaded windows. The cool interior of the ancient cottage urged us outside.

'We'll harvest the far field this morning, All right? You can drive the tractor, John, and would you like to help load the bales of hay, Sally?'

'Yes, I'd love to.' I was ready to do anything. John glanced at me. My smooth pianist's hands were a dead giveaway. I was a novice. Would I be more of a hindrance than a help?

The field was massive. There were already huge rectangular bales of hay strewn in uneven lines throughout the field. John drove the tractor though the open gateway, the empty trailer bouncing precariously across the uneven ground.

Pitchfork in hand, I followed Bill. He stuck the fork into the centre of a bale, lifted it high and dropped it onto the trailer. Another farmhand had clambered onto the trailer, was dragging the bales of hay to the back of the trailer and packing them into a neat pile.

I stuck my pitchfork into the centre of one of the bales on the ground. I had to be quick. The tractor was moving away slowly but surely. It did not stop for anyone. I bent my knees and tried to lift the bale. It was very heavy. With gritted teeth I forced the bale up high and threw it in the direction of the trailer. It made it. I stood puffing with the effort. The straw had scratched my arms. This was going to be hard work.

'Have you ever driven a tractor?' Bill asked, lifting the thermos flask cup to his lips.

'No, but I can drive a car all right.'

'Would you like to drive the tractor for a while?'

'Ooh, yes please.' While I would not admit it, my huffing and puffing had alerted the experienced hands that if they were going to get the harvest in on time, I'd have to have a break from trying to load the trailer.

'I'll show you the pedals.' Bill smiled at his wife, handing her his empty flask, and shepherded me to the tractor. John grinned at us.

By now, the trailer was half full. A farm hand jumped onto the back of the trailer and climbed onto the stack of bales. We were ready.

I sat uneasily in the metal tractor seat. I started the engine and put my foot on the accelerator. Nothing happened. I put my foot more firmly down on the accelerator. The vehicle shot forward.

'Hey!' the farmhand yelled. I looked back to see a pair of heels fly over the back of the trailer. I resolved to drive a little slower.

'It's OK, it's OK,' John shouted to me as I struggled to get the tractor on an even path. 'I'll take over for now.' He was still grinning. I stopped the engine and rapidly slid off the seat. My tractor days were over but no one seemed to mind.

Tired, sunburnt and glowing with the feeling of having accomplished a good day's work, John and I helped feed the pigs. The animals pushed together in rows and rows of pens, squealing raucously after hearing the tractor drive into the farmyard. The stench of the pile of manure at the side of the pens was overwhelming. I screwed up my nose and pretended it did not matter.

In the evening, still smelling of the pig farm, we sat in the sitting room and relaxed, savouring the time for rest. I could still smell pig on John's clothes but I must have got acclimatized to it for it was far more bearable than when I first noticed it. It reminded me of earthier things than the petrol fumes of London I had endured when I had worked there some months before teaching in Peterborough. I nodded to myself; no matter how strong the smell, I preferred John's country smells to those of the city. I did not dare think what my particular perfume was like.

'Let's go for a walk,' he said. A walk? We had only just sat down. He certainly had a lot of energy.

'I'm happy here,' I replied. I thought I had had enough physical activity for the day.

'Come on,' he insisted. Bill and Mary were hovering in the background. They could probably do with some time alone together. I sighed, gave in and out we went.

The sun was just setting and the fresh twilight air was filled with birdsong. I *did* like this tamed country where you could wander out at night without being attacked by mosquitoes and where it was still light at 10p.m.

As we reached the gateway to next door's property John stopped.

'What are we stopping for?' I watched with astonishment as he dropped to the ground.

'What are you doing?' I asked 'Get up.' He was embarrassing me.

'I can only offer myself,' he started, one knee on the ground. Good grief, I thought, he's not going to ask me to marry him, is he?

'Will you marry me?' Well I never. This was a bit sudden. But even though I had known John for only three highly entertaining weeks, I knew that he was the one for me. I should have played the game and made him wait, but I couldn't be bothered.

'Yes,' I spluttered, a little too quickly. We almost danced back to the house to spread the news. I held John's hand as we joyously retraced our steps. I glanced at him. He smiled. The clock had been ticking. I *did* want to get married and have children and at least I could look up to this man. He had charisma. He was the life of the party, cracked jokes, brought out sayings that entertained us all. He knew so much, something about everything. I was fascinated. I should say that the ground moved when we kissed, but to be honest it didn't. There would be time to develop that side of the relationship — at least he was not like the rogues I had known in my university days.

Life would be interesting with John, I thought. I felt there was something more to our very young relationship than I had experienced with anyone else. We seemed to share the same ideals, wanted the same kind of future, had both been hurt and now wanted to make a go of it. For the first time in my life I felt someone really did want me, really loved me in the way that mattered and really wanted to settle down with me. Here was someone I could look up to, I could respect. He may have had slight indigestion problems — he told me it went with his blue eyes and said nothing more. He did have a problem with his mother, but who didn't have a problem with one's mother-in-law? It was to be expected. Even if she tried to break up our relationship I could handle it, couldn't I? I knew for a fact, life would be entertaining with him — there would never be a dull moment.

I telephoned my father. 'Dad, I'm engaged!'

There was a long pause. His pause was much longer than I expected. Did Dad have some reservations about my getting married? Finally, he came out with it. He could stand it no longer. He had to ask:

'What colour?' Poor Dad, he had seen me befriend people from Greece, Spain, and China. He feared above all things that I would marry one of them but he had managed to keep his thoughts to himself. He knew it was wrong to be racially prejudiced and had agreed that one shouldn't let colour or race interfere with relationships, but he couldn't help himself.

I laughed. 'He's British and he's white.' Dad heaved a sigh of relief.

I walked around my room at Mrs Edwards', glowing. I was engaged! I flung myself on the bed and hugged myself. One day soon I would be a married lady; we would have lots of children and maybe live in an old farm house like this. I closed my eyes and pictured John's open face, the slight tilt in his head as he grinned whimsically. I heard a car pull up outside. I slid off the bed and ran to the window. It was John!

I ran downstairs quickly to the door. We hugged and kissed and sat down close together on the sofa in the dark sitting room.

'So how's my girl?' he grinned. I smiled. Where was the ring? Why hadn't John at least mentioned the ring? Did he have cold feet? Did he think he could get away without a ring? I knew John was thrilled, excited, and jovial but I also sensed beneath a dark secret gripping him inside. The shadow of his mother hovered between us. Could he not summon the courage to go against his mother's wishes and seal our promise with a ring? I held my tongue for the moment.

'You know when I told my mother I was going to ask you to marry me,' he confided, 'she told me not to. She said she didn't know anything about you, your family, or where you came from.'

He was sitting close to me, holding my hands. Why had he told me this? There was part of him that was so innocent. It was charming, likeable, and so different from the hardened blokes who had leered over me in the past. If he had any sense, he would not be telling me such things. His honesty was disarming, touching and, I had to admit it, appealing.

'Well, I don't know much about you,' I piped, 'but I know you well enough to trust you. I don't need a pedigree certificate. You are who you are. It's you I'm marrying, not your ancestors nor your mother. Don't worry, she'll come around' He did not look convinced.

'I *would* like you to meet my mother.' His voice was urgent. 'Would you come to ours tomorrow and I'll introduce you?'

I would rather have spent my time with John, alone, but I guessed I was being complimented. After all, we were supposed to be engaged and it was important for his family to meet me.

'I'd love to,' I lied. I tried to imagine a female older version of John. Short? Dark-haired? Bubbly and full of jokes? I could not really picture her.

Chapter 5

The house was an imposing white mansion near the centre of Peterborough. My little Fiat with its streak of oil over its backside looked decidedly out of place.

The door was flung open. John grinned.

'Come in and meet my mother.' He beckoned me inside; his slim shoulders flung back, his face lit up with pride.

The house was dark and cool. It was spotlessly clean; everything was in its place. This was certainly nothing like the creative chaos I lived in as a child and it was certainly nothing like the various places I had inhabited since I had left home. While I tried to be reasonably tidy, there was one aspect of keeping house that I had never really learnt to cope with and that was the cleaning. We had always had a cleaning lady doing that job for us in Tasmania and while my school friends had spent their Saturday mornings cleaning house with their mothers, I usually lay in bed, sleeping in, or I went to town to buy some photography equipment. I could never be accused of being house-proud. As I walked past the glistening laundry sink I wondered if John knew what he was doing. I suspected that his mother and I did not have a lot in common, except perhaps determination and obstinacy. Maybe that's what he saw in us that made him think we were well suited.

My imagined picture of his mother was nothing like the tall, slim, graceful woman who stood before me. We stood apart, embarrassed. No names, no introduction other than John shepherding me closer. He did *so* want us to get on. But the face that turned away from me was so hurt, so tense, there was never going to be any of the warmth I had always felt from my own mother. I looked beyond my future mother-in-law to the mantelpiece. There was a large picture of an older version of John smiling and a picture of her with four other people. I wondered if they were one of her husband and one of her with her brothers and sisters. There was a small chap on the end who looked even more like John than his father. She glared at me, stepped forward and swept past me towards the laundry near the back door. I looked at John. He moved his head sideways beckoning me to follow her. I followed her and found her clutching a shirt, rubbing the collar, lathering it with strong soap with all her force.

'You don't know what it's like,' she moaned. 'I will be all alone. I cook for him, I clean for him.' She scrubbed more furiously. John egged me on further. I forced myself to move towards her. My instinct was to turn back, to leave but I repeated in my head again and again: It is John I am marrying, not his mother. I will not have to live with her and the least I can do is pretend to be willing to extend the olive branch.

I stretched up and put an arm round her shoulders. They were taut, unyielding.

'You're not losing a son, you're gaining a daughter,' I said. She scrubbed harder. We both knew I was not speaking from the heart. It was something to be said to cover the embarrassment. John stood close, fidgeting and anxious.

The figure in the care home bed screwed up his face. He cried. Something had upset him, but what? Was he suddenly aware that he was stuck in this care home bed, never ever to leave, never ever able to walk out a free man or join me as I continued to enjoy life the way we used to have together? It would be better if he were never aware of his predicament or his surroundings. Why was life so cruel? Or worse still, did he know by instinct what I was thinking? I could never share my thoughts about his mother with him. He never fully understood my feelings or why there would always be a rift between his mother and me. His mother was unhappy, and no amount of pleading and persuading would bring her round. But she needed him desperately, or was it that John needed her desperately? If so, why?

I patted John's hand. 'It's all right. You're all right. I'm here. There's nothing to cry about.' My heart wrenched. His contorted face seemed to say that he knew he was a prisoner in this distorted body. Yes, he *was* suddenly aware of just how much he was suffering. Would it be better that he had no idea, or that he was aware of what was going on? I did not let myself think of what I could have wished for. The future would be whatever it would be.

'What more could you want?' My tone was light, masking my true feelings. 'You have a comfortable bed, your loving wife by your side. You have the hot and cold nurses you always wanted, haven't you?' I kept trying to put a lift into my voice to cheer him up but my stomach gripped. He used to grin broadly every time I teased him in this way before, but this time, this time he was blank. The tears had stopped and the contorted face eased a little, but there was no smile, no light in the eyes. A chance stream of sunlight flashed into the room. The classical music played on.

I sat back in the chair allowing myself to daydream.

The classical music the school orchestra played at Peak Lane Comprehensive School in Peterborough was not quite up to the standard that was playing in John's room, but it came quite close. I was teaching at the school when I became engaged. As I marched down the corridors, acting as though I had all the confidence in the world, I could hear excited twittering behind me as I passed a group of staring students.

One of the students muttered just loud enough so that I could hear but not loud enough so that I could accuse him of being disrespectful, 'I thought she was supposed to be engaged. So where's the ring?'

I wondered that too. When I met John that night I decided to confront him.

'Are we really engaged? Are we getting a ring?' I blurted as he sat down on the sofa. 'It's getting difficult to convince people that we are really engaged without a ring to show for it, you know.'

He looked troubled, confused. I felt guilty immediately but it was no good, we were engaged or we were not engaged and a ring was a must. I sat next to him leaned forward and looked at him. 'We could go into town tomorrow straight after work. You could make it then, couldn't you?'

'I guess so. Mother —' He decided against finishing the sentence, looked into my eyes and held my hand. 'Yes. Of course, I'll pick you up at the school gate at 4 p.m.'

The little jeweller's shop was in the High Street of Peterborough. Dark wood contrasted with spotlights blazing on rows of sparkling diamonds. Would I ask for the biggest diamond I could see?

'May I see the most expensive one you have?' I asked, glancing at John. He did not even blink. The jeweller brought a large diamond ring for me to peruse.

'Mm, lovely, but it's a bit showy for me. What about a medium-priced one with a couple of small diamonds?' Again John did not flinch. 'This one will do nicely.' I looked at John, seeking approval. He nodded.

I chose a gold ring with a central sapphire with two small diamonds either side. It fitted beautifully. I stood back giving John space on the counter to write the cheque. At last!

We left the shop together. I put my hand on John's arm, displaying the ring for all to see. The world was rosy and I had a wonderful future to look forward to.

As we walked to his car, I said. 'Let's get married soon — say in a few months. What about October?'

'Mother says October is not a good month. It's Autumn, there might be rain. '

'November?'

'No fruits, no flowers, No-vember. She says that's not a good month either.'

'December?'

'Mother says that's too near Christmas.'

So he and his mother had already been discussing when we would get married. Whose marriage was it? I sat on the settee, next to John, moving the ring up and down my finger. Maybe if I was going to change my mind, this was the time to do it.

John sensed my uneasiness. 'Look,' he said, putting his arm around me. 'Why not wait until next year to give your father enough time to arrange his trip. You do want your father at the wedding, don't you?'

I nodded. My bottom lip pushed forward I said, 'Well then, when?'

'Why not February? That will give your father plenty of time to organize his trip. I know it is the rainiest month of the year and we call it "February fill-dyke", but the sun can shine in February. I will tell Mother. She will have to accept it.'

February it was then.

'Meanwhile, let's enjoy ourselves. Let's go out tomorrow,' he said.

'Where to?' I asked cagily. Not to Mother's again, I hoped.

'I'll take you out to lunch, for a surprise. I know you'll like it.'

I could not contain myself any longer. 'Will we be picking up your mother first?' I could not bring myself to call her 'Mother' yet and 'Eunice' just did not seem to be appropriate. We had never discussed what I should call her.

'No, Mother will be going to a friend's for the day,' John said grimly.

'Will she?' I said, trying not to look too pleased. So she did have friends, after all. Why did she have to have her son at her every beck and call then? And why was John so grim about it? Surely he should be delighted that he would be free from her for one day, at least?

After a long night, the morning finally dawned. I was excited. At last we were going out together for the whole day, alone. His white Ford Escort swept into the yard. There was someone sitting next to him. John stepped out of the car quickly.

'I've brought Mother too, I hope you don't mind?' My heart shrank. Of course I minded but complaining was not going to help matters. I climbed into the back seat and said nothing. John drove along very narrow, bumpy roads. His mother sat stiffly in the front seat next to him.

I noticed that at times we overlooked the fields. They were much lower than I expected. As if reading my thoughts, John said, 'I thought you would like to see something of the Fens first. The fields around us have been drained so the land has shrunk. That's why the roads are higher and you will see that even the rivers are higher here.' He steadied the wheel as the car leapt over an unexpectedly large bump. He nodded towards a village church. 'That's called the Pepper pot.'

As he described what we were seeing, his voice had the same richness that I had first noticed and liked, but there was a tinge of darkness about his words. It was as though he was speaking automatically to an unknown tourist. Something was bothering him. I shrugged my shoulders. It might have been the fact that his mother was with him. I would worry about that later. His mother sighed. I looked towards the village on the hill with its unusual church. The tower was squat, and yes, it looked exactly like a pepper pot. I loved English eccentricities. Glancing at John's strong face in the mirror as he concentrated on negotiating the narrow road, I wondered if his own brand of eccentricity, his darker side, his hidden troubles, were attracting me. His mother coughed into the back of her hand.

'Don't drive too fast,' she snapped. John pursed his lips.

We drove along another long, narrow and bumpy road surrounded by lower fields. I read the next village sign.

'What a strange name, Earith.'

'Yes it means dweller at the gravel harbour.' John changed down a gear.

'Is there a gravel harbour here?'

'No, someone would have come from a gravel harbour, probably in Kent and given his name to the place he settled — Earith.'

'Ah, so nothing to do with ears then?'

''Fraid not,' John grinned. 'See those large empty fields on either side of the road now?' He jerked his head to the right.

'Yes.' A cow was lethargically pulling at the thin grass.

'That's where they let the rivers flood when there is too much water. I'll bring you here in winter sometime. It's spectacular.'

'I hope it's not too long before we have lunch,' said his mother icily.

I decided to ignore her and asked 'What's the name of the river, John?'

'The Great Ouse.'

'There's a river Ouse in Tasmania. I've noticed that a lot of our names have been borrowed from

England. I saw on the map there is even a Devonport in England.'

'Yes, well, we've got to give the colonies something.' He glanced into the mirror and winked at me, his blue eyes twinkling with mischief. Then he became more serious. 'There are two more rivers here, the Old and New Bedford Rivers. One of them, the New Bedford River, or Hundred Foot Drain, is man-made. It was built between Earith and Denver Sluice to take the excess water. It's tidal, and at Welney you can see how they've made the river flow backwards some 30 miles from the sea.'

'Wow' I said. It seemed so much trouble for such a small area of land. 'I suppose the population being what it is, it was worth all that trouble.'

'Indeed.'

A sign for Needingworth appeared.

'Here's another strange name,' I said. 'Why on earth would they call a place "Needingworth"? I'm not sure I'd like to live in a place called that.'

'The place we are going to is called Holywell, which derived its name from a spring of fresh water there. One of my uncles had a farm there once. It could have been mine ...' He bit his lip.

'Yours? You could have been a farmer here?'
His mother glared at him quickly. 'Watch what you're doing!' she snapped as he narrowly missed a pigeon on the road.

He did not answer my question. The atmosphere in the car was electric. He closed his lips firmly and turned the wheel to sweep round the corner a little faster that I would have liked. I gripped the seat.

'We're nearly there.' His voice had returned to the matter-of-fact, isn't-this-interesting tone.

'I should think so,' his mother snapped.

'We'll have lunch at the oldest inn in the country,' John continued in a calmer tone. 'It's called the Old Ferry Boat Inn.' He changed gear again as we went round another corner, at a sensible pace this time. 'It was built in Anglo-Saxon times, and it's said that alcohol was sold here as early as 560 BC.' He grinned. 'I think they've changed the barrels since then.'

'Ha ha', I forced a laugh. He really could be corny at times, but what did it matter? At least he was trying to be cheerful again. His mother remained impassively in her seat and said nothing.

The Old Ferry Boat Inn sat firmly in a picture-postcard scene. The large building was heavily covered with a thick thatched roof and had solid smooth white walls. Lush green grass surrounded it. The river ambled by in a lazy curve.

'It's lovely!' I exclaimed.

John broke into a smile, drove the car into the car park and pulled up. He leapt out of the car swiftly, opened his mother's door and waited patiently while she slowly stepped out. I was determined to make sure he opened my door too. I turned my gaze away from his mother's glare.

'Thank you, kind sir,' I said to John after he had opened my door. It felt good climbing out of the car while my handsome fiancé waited, even though my ungainly manner was nothing like the smooth graceful movements of his mother. I tried to ignore the unhappy figure of his mother waiting impatiently for me to join her.

Chapter 6

The sun shone brightly on the inn, making the stark white walls sparkle as if to greet us. We entered the building and inside the door I paused for a moment, taking in the atmosphere. Large hand-hewn oak beams framed the walls. I wondered why our Tasmanian houses were made of simple overlapping wooden planks. If they could build places like this in England centuries before Tasmania was first colonized, why not continue? I did not remember seeing any properties like this in Tasmania, not with oak beams as big as this.

'It's beautiful.' I turned to John. He beamed as if it was all his own doing. I put my arm into his, making sure my engagement ring was in full view as we joined his mother inside.

'I'm not hungry anymore,' she blurted. We stared at her. She grimaced and led the way into the darkness.

'Let's sit near the window' I said, moving towards an empty table bathed in sunlight.

'No, we will sit by the picture over there,' his mother barked.

'Now, now ladies,' John chuckled. 'I will make the decision, and we will sit in the centre of the room just here.' He held a chair back. I waited while his mother sat down. It was too much to expect for John to look after me first.

Our conversation was polite, stilted and cold. The meal lost much of its taste as far as I was concerned for I had to fight back the bile that was filling my mouth and my thoughts.

'I think I will powder my nose,' said John's mother as she stood up and turned to go towards the ladies' room.

'I will too,' I said to John and followed smartly behind her.

I waited until she was just inside the door.

'I need a word with you,' I said menacingly in her ear while her back was turned to me.

She turned around, shocked at my tone.

'And, young lady, who do you think you are to take that tone with me?'

'Whether you like it or not, John and I are getting married,' I flung my wrist up at her face so that the engagement ring almost touched her nose.

She pushed my hand away. 'He is still my son, my only son,' she snarled. 'Who do you think you are coming into our lives and spoiling everything?'

'I'm someone who cares about John and not just myself,' I snapped.

'If you really cared about him, you wouldn't have agreed to marry him,' she said.

'That's what you would have wanted, isn't it? It would not matter who he married — anyone he married would be wrong for him. You just want him for yourself.' My voice was rising, my words tripping over themselves. 'You will have to stop all this nastiness, and treat me as an equal or you are going to have an even harder time of it than you're having now.'

'That's what you think. John knows where his place is. Your marriage won't last a month, I'll see to that.' She pulled away from me. 'That's if you get married at all!' she snarled as she went into a cubicle.

I stood back, stunned. Where were all her tears now? Her eyes had been wild with anger, but there was not a tear in sight and I had seen so many of those when John had insisted on calling at her house whenever we went out in Peterborough.

The following weekend John and I were sitting close together on the sofa, holding hands. I had not told John of the argument his mother and if he knew about it, he was tactful enough not to mention it. He turned to me.

'There's a walk for charity next week — 25 miles.'

'Yes?'

'Mother thinks it would be a lovely idea if we went on it. Mother gives to that charity ever since Uncle Jim ...' He stopped abruptly and glanced at me quickly hoping I had not heard his last slip of the tongue. He obviously did not want me to know about Uncle Jim, whoever he was. I didn't care. I was marrying John, not his family. He said quickly 'We'll go.'

We will? I thought. I had never been on a 5-mile charity walk, let alone a 25-mile one. Did his mother have an instinct for things I did not like? Was this one of her tests? Who was Uncle Jim and what was the charity? Well, whatever the charity and whatever there was to learn about Uncle Jim, I would go if I wanted to and would stay at home if I decided it was not for me. It certainly was not for *her* to decide. To be on the safe side, I feigned interest. It wouldn't hurt me to go on a twenty-five-mile walk, would it? I should support my fiancé in all things, shouldn't I? The thought filled me with dread. It was the last thing I really wanted to do after a week of jostling with a hundred or so hormonally driven teenagers. Well, what harm would it do? Then on the Thursday, I sneezed. A cold! I had come down with a cold. Wonderful! I was far too ill to go on such a long walk.

'I'b sorry,' I mumbled into the phone, 'I canno cub on de wal. I'b too ill. Cab you go ob your owb? You'll be all righ, won' you?'

The day after the walk, a bow-legged figure struggled towards to door of Mrs Edwards'.

'It was wonderful!' he grinned. 'I made it!' He strained to lift his feet over the threshold.

'You look awfully stiff. Your Uncle Jim will be proud of you.' I stood up quickly leaving a space for him to flop down. 'Sit down.'

John sat down on the sofa awkwardly. 'It was a tremendous experience. You should have come you know.' He paused. 'And I think you should forget about Uncle Jim. You have nothing to gain from knowing about him. Forget him. I don't want you to mention him again.' He scowled and looked directly into my eyes. I feigned a neutral expression. There would be time for Uncle Jim when John was ready.

'We raised a lot of money for a worthy cause,' he said, rubbing his leg. 'You know, when I was at school, my friend and I would cycle to Hunstanton and back, some fifty miles or so.'

'All that way? Wow!' I was impressed. Was I marrying some kind of fitness freak? Well, no matter. I could never be accused of being freakish about exercise.

I avoided it when possible and maybe I would be able to calm his frantic energy into something more normal. Opposites attract, they say.

The wedding day grew closer and Dad was coming early to enjoy a long holiday and to stay for the wedding.

The drive to Heathrow Airport was long and tedious, but there was a feeling of delicious expectation in us. We were going to meet my dad.

'That's him!' John said, as a stream of people came out of the exit.

'No, that's nothing like him,' I said, scathingly. 'How could you possibly recognize him? You have never even met him. I know my dad and that is not my dad.'

The figure in the large hat came towards us. As he got closer his features became clearer.

I rushed towards him. 'Oh my gosh! It *is* Dad after all.' I gave him a big hug.

John gripped his hand firmly. 'Welcome to England.'

I beamed.

As the wedding day grew closer, Dad and I went out together for a last father-daughter meal before the big day when I was to become a married lady.

'Well, you've still got time to change your mind,' Dad smiled at me.

'No, I won't be doing that.' I grinned awkwardly. Sometimes Dad's humour really did annoy me.

'John's mother seems very pleasant,' he said, looking at me intently.

'Does she?' I bit my lip. How could he not see what she was really like? I looked at his open Aussie countenance. He did not have a nasty bone in his body. He would never see, or be allowed to see, the other side of the woman who was to be my mother-in-law. I decided to hold my tongue. He would find out soon enough.

My father fingered his coffee cup. 'You know,' he said, pausing slightly, 'John's a little unusual.' He obviously sensed something not quite right, something different, about John.

'I know,' I snapped, 'but my brother is pretty unusual and he's basically OK. Right?'

Dad did not reply.

We had been to the little church in Peterborough and had the banns read three weeks in a row. No one had interrupted the service to announce that there was a reason why we could not get married. I had expected his mother to come storming down the aisle demanding a rethink, but no, she was much too graceful, much more subtle than that. I glanced at John. Could it possibly be that John had secretly married before? After all, there were hidden depths to his life and secrets in his family that he was reluctant to reveal. When I asked questions I always felt I was not being given the whole story. However, if I had been asked such searching questions, I too, would probably have fobbed them off with vague replies.

'There's many a slip twixt cup and lip,' John chirped when we joked about whether one of us would not turn up at the wedding. The ghost of his previous fiancée lay between us.

One evening, as we relaxed in the softened light of the sitting room, I turned to John and asked, point blank, 'Do you mind telling me why you didn't marry your first fiancée?'

He paused, a wistful look flashed in his eyes, a look that for a split second suggested regret.

'There was something not right about our relationship,' John said, fingering his tie. 'There was something wrong with her health but she wouldn't tell me what it was. She went to hospital and had tests, but still would not tell me.'

'For better or worse, though, isn't it?'

'There was more. Her father owned the village shop and I would have been expected to serve in it. I would have ended up a slave to her father. I wanted my independence.' He looked at the floor. 'Besides, it was too soon after my father had died. It was only six weeks to the wedding date. It was too soon. Mother ...' His voice trailed off. I would get no more from him that night.

It was now six weeks before our wedding date. I felt very uneasy. He had called off the wedding six weeks before he was supposed to marry his precious fiancée — he might do the same to me. He must have been mad to call it off so late in the piece — or brave. I decided on the latter. Would he do it again?

Chapter 7

The six weeks turned into two and we were soon sitting in front of the vicar for our pep talk.

'If you have any misgivings, now is the time to speak them.' The vicar's voice resonated in the vicarage sitting room. 'You should trust each other without question.' His fatherly tones lay suspended in the silence.

I looked down. I could trust John; trust him to make things interesting, difficult and maybe a challenge to deal with. I had long decided that love was definitely not blind, but real love was knowing your partner very well, faults and all; real love was being ready and able to deal with the faults that you both had. After all, I was hardly one to complain. My brother's first comment when he knew we were getting married was that I was a lucky person to find anyone to take me on.

I trusted John to be honourable and to do the best he could, but would this be good enough? He still needed his mother in a way that a man of his age should have long outgrown. Could I trust him to leave his mother and allow our relationship to grow?

I looked up. I should speak now but I couldn't. I decided that I would take the risk. I felt strong enough to cope for the both of us.

16th February 1974, the day of the wedding, arrived. Like all major events in my life, I treated it as another 'ordinary' day, something to be lived through. I felt a bit like a turkey dressed for the kill but I put those thoughts aside.

'Oh my goodness,' Mrs Edwards said in excitement. She was more excited than I was. 'I do need to vacuum the hallway.'

'I'll do it, I'll do it,' I said hurriedly. I had never bothered to vacuum the hallway before, but now it was different. Quickly I grabbed the vacuum cleaner and dashed up and down the hallway. I finished by wrapping the cord hurriedly around the handle.

'I must get into my dress now,' I said, rushing upstairs before she had anything else to panic about.

I held onto Dad's arm and walked along the path to the church, my wedding dress flicking my uncomfortable white shoes as the cool sun smiled weakly. 'Here comes the bride, fair fat and wide' echoed in my mind as we walked up the aisle. Was his mother there, or was she missing? She had threatened John so many times that she was not going to come. I pushed the thought out of my mind and concentrated on looking happy, not dropping the flowers and watching my feet while I tried at the same time to hold my head high. I wish I had thought of some less stereotyped music for my entry. I dared not look at the vicar. What if John wasn't there?

Then I saw him, waiting for me. He grinned broadly, his body rigid with nerves. His hand clammy as I held it.

'We are gathered together ...' the vicar's calm words began the service. We had made it!

With a slight tremble in our voices, we said 'I do' and the panic was over. I had the ring on my finger and all we had to do now was sign the register. The organist played Pachelbel's Canon — just the right kind of quiet calming music, I thought, as we made our way to the table. We posed as we pretended to sign, our photograph was taken, again and again and finally I signed the register properly. Then it was John's turn. He pressed the pen down hard. I heard a snap. John grinned sheepishly.

'I'm sorry; I seem to have broken the pen.'

'The pen? Broken?' This was new for even this seasoned vicar. 'I think there is another one in the vestry.' In a flurry of gown, the vicar disappeared for a few moments and swept back again, holding another pen. He gave it to John saying

'Perhaps you should not press so hard this time?' John fumbled for a moment and finally managed to add his signature. At last we walked down the aisle triumphantly as the organist struggled valiantly to play Widor's Fifth Toccata on the tiny church organ. We were married!

At the lunch at the Gordon Arms Hotel, Dad stood up and started his speech. I looked at the guests. John had insisted that we only have my dad and his mother as family representatives. As Dad was paying, I did not argue. Still, my school buddies smiled warmly. Mary and Bill beamed at me. They were as good as family, I supposed.

'She was a very quiet baby ...' my dad began. I hid my head. Did he really have to bring this up?

'We were about to go to bed one night and thought we had forgotten something. Suddenly we realized we had left the baby outside. We had forgotten all about her!' I thought to myself what a different person I had grown into from what the behaviour of the baby in his story might have suggested. I smiled politely. Dad was doing his best.

We said goodbye to everyone and I let John have a last poignant moment with his mother, who was weeping into an embroidered hanky. He finally managed to calm her down. He opened the car door for her, kissed her one last time and the driver smoothly drove the car away. I heaved a sigh of relief.

We changed into our going-away clothes and sped towards our first night of the honeymoon at the University Arms Hotel in Cambridge.

The spires of Cambridge greeted us as John drove us towards the centre of the city. He turned into the car park beneath the University Arms Hotel and, feeling like royalty, we climbed out and went to the reception desk. The staff grinned at us. There was no hiding our reason for being there.

We walked up the carpeted stairs, so wide, so plush. It was wonderful. John unlocked the door and we stepped in. There was a TV in the room — luxury, sheer luxury! I turned and looked out of the window. Stretching beneath us were the stripes of a beautifully mown lawn, nothing like the straggly blanched grass heads of the lawns in Tasmania.

We really were in Cambridge, the hallowed city of learning that I had always wanted to visit. Now, I was really here, not as a stranger but as a married woman — a real live *married* woman, married to an Englishman. Wonderful. We would soon have children and our lives would be fulfilled. I'd made it!

'No need for contraception,' I laughed.

'I think we ought to wait a while before we have children.'

'But I thought we would have them straight away? That's why we got married, isn't it?'

'I really think we ought to wait.' It was no good arguing; I knew that it was important to follow John's wishes more than my own if our relationship was to work. Part of me rebelled but I instinctively knew that it would be fatal to push John into a direction he did not want to follow. He wanted to wait before we had children, so I would have to wait. I paused. Maybe he was right after all; for we needed to make sure we got along together well enough when we lived in the same house at close quarters. Besides, a little more time might reveal what lay behind John's mysterious background. So we waited.

While the earth did not move for me on our first night, it was every bit a first night in all other senses. We breakfasted like a couple from an Agatha Christie novel, seated at the linen-clothed table, with a choice for a cooked breakfast. John paid the bill; we climbed into the car and drove to the airport to catch our flight to Majorca. I was excited.

'I've never been to Majorca before. I wonder if it's like Barcelona?' I smiled at John as he drove. He did not reply. He was concentrating on his driving. I sat back in my seat. After several miles I spoke again.

'I believe the composer Chopin used to live on the island of Majorca. Do you think we'll see the place where he lived?'

Still John did not reply. His eyes remained focused on the road ahead. I settled down in the seat again and allowed myself to daydream.

I was at the piano, playing Chopin's 'Revolutionary Study'. I could feel the crashing right hand chords under my fingers and I revelled in the thunderous runs in the left hand. Chopin knew how to feel pain and anger. He knew what passion, real passion, was about. What would his house be like? Would I see the piano he used and maybe some of his music? Would I be able to conjure up just how he felt as he composed music that reached the very depths of the soul? He knew how it was to suffer. I glanced at my left hand. Yes, the wedding ring was still there. It felt large and chunky on my hand.

'So, we are licensed now, John,' I tried for a third time. I looked at him. He was smiling this time. He looked as fresh-faced and euphoric as I was. We were a couple of glowing newlyweds. Chopin would have to take second place today. I had other things to think about and enjoy.

At last we were in our hotel in Majorca. Music was playing in the background. 'Viva España,' I joined in the chorus enthusiastically.

'Isn't this great?' I grinned at John.

He smiled absently in return. 'I hope we can get an English newspaper soon,' he said, making for the door. 'I'll go and ask for one at the desk.' Left on my own in the small hotel room, I grimaced: the wretched election. Surely our marriage was more important than any event way back in England? Whatever happened, there was nothing he could do about it, so why couldn't he wait until we got back?

I waited for my new husband to return, to look dreamily into my eyes and to plan our wonderful days of honeymooning. Instead, he came back clutching the newspaper and proceeded to read it cover to cover.

'So much for my charm,' I muttered, lying next to him, trying to remember every line of his face. He did not reply.

After several days during which I felt very neglected, John finally swept into the room triumphantly one morning. 'We won!' he shouted. 'The Conservatives are in!'

'Bully for them,' I said, trying not to show the annoyance I felt. At least his mother had been left out of the conversation for a while. I grinned. Now to the honeymoon, I thought.

We had finished cleaning our teeth after breakfast the next morning. I flopped onto the bed and asked, 'What would you like to do today: walk through the streets, go shopping, take a trip into the countryside?'

'Nothing.' John sat stiffly in the chair.

'Come on, let's do something now. Let's go for a walk.' I stood up and pulled his hand.

'No, I want to stay here.' He sat staring out of the window at the tall dark green palms.

'Come on. Don't be a spoilsport.' I tried to keep the tone light. 'Let's go into town and have a look around.'

John spoke through gritted teeth. 'No!'

'Come on,' I pleaded. 'You'll enjoy it.'

'No!' He was decidedly angry this time.

'Can you hear that song again?' I joined in the chorus to 'Viva España'. 'That could be our song. I want to buy a record of it. Shall I?'

'No!'

'Why not? What's the matter? What is it?'

He did not reply. I tried to encourage him to explore with me. He would have none of it. He wanted to stay in the hotel. There was obviously something troubling him deeply but I convinced myself that it was nothing that we couldn't overcome. I shrugged. One day I would find out what demon was stifling him. Given time and my wonderful care he would soon be healed of this spectre that haunted him.

I grabbed my key to the room.

'Well, if you want to stay and sulk, you can. I'm going out on my own to explore. I'll be back sometime.' John looked blankly at me. 'Okay? Change your mind?' John did not move. He turned his face away from me.

I flung open the door, swept outside and shut the door firmly behind me. I walked quickly down the hall without looking back. I would not be upset by John's behaviour.

Chapter 8

I walked a short distance from the hotel. The warm sun in February, the lush green tropical plants and the sound of voices speaking a foreign tongue were enough to cheer me. I looked at the expensive clothes and accessories in the shop windows. I came across a music shop at the end of the street. I went in and fingered through the records. I found a copy of 'Viva España'. The cover was bright, inviting, the words 'Viva España' in bold across the top. How I wanted a copy! I pulled it out glanced towards the salesperson but hesitated. What would be wrong with buying a single copy of this record? Why was John so against it? I sighed, replacing the record amongst the others. There was not much point in upsetting John more than he was already. I went outside into the bright sunshine.

When I returned to our room John stood up as I bounced inside.

'I had a great time. It's gorgeous out there. It is so lovely to be able to walk in the sunshine in February of all months. I think I want to learn Spanish one day.'
He pulled me to him and held onto me as though he never wanted to let me go. But still he said nothing.

We walked into the dining room for dinner that night as though nothing untoward had happened in our day. I forced a smile at the couple who were sitting next to us.

'Are you on honeymoon too?' John asked them.

'Why, yes,' the young man replied, his curly brown hair bobbing as he spoke. 'I'm Owen and this is my wife Lynn.' He spoke with a London accent. 'It's a great hotel isn't it?' His light blue eyes sparkled.

'Yes, it is indeed,' said John. 'As the great Oscar Wilde said: "I have the simplest tastes. I am always satisfied with the best." I'm John,' John's hand reached for mine 'and this is my wife, Sally.' His voice cracked with pride.

I smiled and relaxed. At last the old John was back, but how long would he stay like this? Had I married a new Jekyll and Hyde? I refused to worry about it now.

John continued, 'How long are you staying?'

'We're going tomorrow,' Lynn said looking down at her untouched soup.

'Oh, what a pity', I said. 'We've got a few more days yet.' I smiled at her, hoping I had disguised the unease I still felt.

Owen turned his head quickly towards me. 'That's an interesting accent. Where do you come from? No, no,' he stopped me before I could speak again. 'Let me guess. New Zealand?'

'No!' I grimaced, 'not New Zealand. You offend me, kind sir,' I joked. 'I come from Australia, Tasmania to be exact.'

'Ah, Australia, the land of wide open spaces and gold, pots of gold.'

'Why do you say "pots of gold"? I don't think it has any more than other countries, California, for a start.'

'Oh, it's just that I remember my mother getting postcards from a place in Australia where there was gold — was it Ben something?'

'Bendigo?'

'Yeah, that's right. My ma's aunt had shocked the family by having an affair with a married man. I believe they ran off to Australia and made it rich in the goldfields of Bendigo.'

John fidgeted in his seat. 'Where is that waitress?' he asked, stretching his body to scan the restaurant.

'So you must be very wealthy then?'

'Ah no, no such luck. The chap dumped my aunt as soon as they arrived — before he found a huge nugget of gold. He gave all of his wealth to his children. Ma's poor aunt became the barmaid at the local pub. Ma always had a good laugh when her postcards arrived, she told such good stories. She did hate her ex-lover though, Cocky Cox she called him.'

Cox? I sat up. I searched my memory. I thought Mary had mentioned the name when she had talked about John's aunts. I turned sharply to the speaker 'Cox? That's ...' I felt a sharp pain on my ankle. John glared at me. I raised my eyebrows. 'That's an interesting name,' I finished, looking down at my empty plate. What was the problem with John now? I decided not to ask him directly. Give him time and he would tell me.

'Waitress!' John called and a slim young girl, her face flushed, rushed to the table.

Back in the hotel room, I turned to John.

'It was an interesting couple we met tonight,' I commented, testing John's mood.

'Yes,' he said glumly, looking out the window.

'Why did you kick me when Owen said the name Cox?'

'I didn't want you to say my mother's surname. It's nothing to do with them. You never know with complete strangers,' John flushed. We both knew he was lying. I decided to leave it alone for the moment.

'Shall we go and see Chopin's place tomorrow?' I asked quickly. 'There is a tour leaving at ten in the morning.' My eyes were steely. John knew that if he did not come, I would be going without him. He hesitated.

'All right then, we'll go. I'll go and book the tickets.' We went down to the reception desk and I stood by his side, proud that my man was at last taking part in this adventure of ours.

In the packed bus, my blouse stuck to me in the heat, but I did not care. John's features remained unmoved and he ignored the drops of sweat forming on his forehead. The bus climbed slowly up into the mountains and the perspiration on my forehead cooled at last. Dark green foliage hid most of the jagged peaks we could see in front. Valleys dropped down beside us. I leaned towards the window peering down. I could not see where they ended. I felt giddy. I decided not to look any more.

'We're here!' the bus driver shouted as he pulled on the handbrake. 'Be back in 2 hours,' he said and opened the bus door.

I was one of the first to scramble off the bus. John followed behind waiting while I absorbed what I could see. We followed the trail of tourists into Chopin's retreat.

The subdued light and shadows on the yellowing keys of the piano transported me into the famous composer's time. I could see his long fingers racing over the keys, dwelling on timeless, poignant melodies. I imagined his soul mate George Sand standing next to him empathizing with his emotional, almost spiritual, outpouring. In my imagination I could hear one of his nocturnes floating into the night air. My soul was transported, soothed by the experience. John remained at my side, curious but unaffected. I sighed and shrugged my shoulders, taking one last look at the tiny room and tempting piano, and made my way back to the bus with John.

Back in the hotel, John snapped.

'I don't know what you saw in it. It was just a room.'

'What an awful thing to say. It was more than just a room. It was history. Chopin is one of our best composers. I wish I could compose like he did. You say you like classical music. Why couldn't you appreciate our visit to his retreat?'

'All they were after was our money. And they got it, too. There are so many gullible people out there willing to part with their shekels to look at a pile of wood and an old piano. You fell for it too.' The horrible John was back. In a numb, dream-like state I held my tongue. One day we would dissipate the wretched malevolence that haunted him.

On the way down to dinner that evening John rushed to the reception desk

'Do you have an English paper?' he asked.

'Yes, sir, here is today's English newspaper, Mr Wilks.' John took the newspaper, sat in one of the chairs nearby and pored over the headlines. I sat next to him, people watching.

'It's going to be a great time for the Conservatives,' he said. 'Did you know ...' he started repeating the news to me. I nodded absently from time to time. At least he was in a better mood now.

Our unique honeymoon was finally over. I sat next to John in the car as he drove towards Peterborough. In a few days I would be back in the packed classroom with a large group of highly charged teenagers to entertain.

We were both bathing in the euphoria of the freshness, the newness of our joint venture. The last time we were in this car we had driven to our honeymoon. Confetti lay on the carpet under our feet. I put my hand on John's slim thigh. He was my man. I was married. I would have someone who would look after me for the rest of my life. I felt cosy, warm, and secure.

'I wonder what my mother has left us in the flat?' John pressed his foot down further on the accelerator. It was three in the morning. The road was perfectly clear. Why did he have to bring his mother into it? I loved my dad dearly, but the last thing I would want him to do was to prepare our flat for us when we came back from our honeymoon. I dozed.

Suddenly my eyes shot open. I peered into the mirror. Another car was behind us. It was speeding towards us, getting closer and closer. John pulled the car over.

'What's the matter?' I shook my head, forcing myself to wake up properly.

'It's a police car.' John put on the hand brake. A policeman tapped on John's window. John wound down the window.

'What's up, officer?' John sounded almost pleased to see him.

'Might I ask what you are doing at this hour in the morning, sir?' I was glad John was doing the talking. I wanted to snap 'None of your business!' but I held my tongue.

'We are returning from our honeymoon,' John said in a proud, matter-of-fact voice.

'May I ask you names, please?'

'John Wilks,' John said, and with a touch of pride in his voice, 'and this is my wife, Sally.'

'Wilks?' He made a note on his pad. His partner joined him.

'Yes. Why do you ask?'

'Oh, it's just that it is rare to see people out at this hour of the morning, sir, and we like to check.' He turned and showed his partner the note on his pad. The partner stared hard at John and shook his head.

'Ah, yes,' the first policeman said. 'I can see the confetti. Thank you, sir. You may go on your way.'
I glanced at John.

'Why do you think they really stopped us?' I looked in the rear vision mirror. The two policemen were still watching us.

'I've no idea,' said John, as he turned the key and the car pulled away.

'He seemed interested in the name "Wilks". Why is that do you think?' I could see the policeman making a note of the number plate.

'My father and the Wilks family are quite famous, you know.' John changed gear.

'Because of your father's finance business?'

'Amongst other reasons, yes.' John closed his mouth firmly, stared ahead and sped forward.

I leaned back. I was too tired to ask any more questions. His father was famous? I would have to look him up in the local newspapers. What next? I had never been stopped and questioned by the police before. Yes, it is definite, life will never be dull with John and he will be my rock against all difficulty, I thought. I leaned back in the passenger's seat and grinned. I was happy. I put all thoughts of the flat and what his mother had done to it behind me.

Chapter 9

As we drove towards the centre of Peterborough, my spirits rose as I increasingly felt we would be in the centre of a very important city, a city full of tradition, a history of fine industry and values — values that would be far bigger and stronger than the petty angst our tiny family endured.

'Here it is.' John led me up the path to the solid-brick, Victorian semi-detached building. I pursed my lips when we went inside. How lovely it would have been if we had stepped into a Victorian world with grand pieces of antique furniture, shiny mahogany, large original paintings and an aspidistra on a solid stand in the hall. Instead, we were met with the post-war fifties and sixties style: cheap, shiny, beige linoleum, and flying ducks above the mantelpiece. I smiled at John. It did not matter that it was unfashionable and that I did not especially like its decor. It was ours, ours alone. We would now have a chance. His mother's touches were no doubt there, but I could not see them and, most importantly, I could not feel them.

In a daze, we unpacked. I was overtired. I knew I would not sleep. I put the kettle on to boil.

'Cup of tea?' I asked. John nodded. He watched while I picked up the kettle.

'You know,' he said, as though thinking aloud, 'my mother did not want us to get married.' I remained silent. He continued, 'She suggested we live together first.'

'Really?' I swirled some of the boiling water round in the teapot and tipped it out into the sink. Maybe I had misjudged her. I had assumed her restrictive personality would mean that she would have none of this modern living-together lark.

'Maybe she hoped that if we lived together we would have too many rows and we would not get married at all in the end,' I suggested.

It was John's turn to remain silent. I put three teaspoons of tea into the pot and filled it with boiling water. The cups and saucers rattled as I placed them on the kitchen table.

'Do you think it has brewed yet?' I asked.

'No, leave it for a bit. I'll pour it when it's ready.'

I leaned my head on my hands. I was so tired.

Months passed and a semblance of normality developed in our daily lives. Part of this was an almost-daily telephone conversation John had with his mother, the arguments becoming more and more heated. Sometimes when he came home from work he would give me a hurried peck on the cheek and grab his keys saying, 'I've got to go to Mother's. She's beside herself. Don't keep any dinner for me, I'll probably eat there.'

Sitting alone in the cold flat, I stirred my tea and contemplated our situation. Peterborough was too close to her. It was too easy for John to run to her every time she called. We needed to move out of the city for the sake of our marriage. I had soon learned that it was no good criticizing her. While I knew that my barbed comments reflected how John felt too, he would never admit it. As her only son, it was his duty to be loyal but he also had a duty to be loyal to me. Poor chap, he was piggy in the middle. We had to do something about it.

One Thursday, the sun streamed into the flat and John came home from work smiling. Now was the time.

'You know,' I said, as casually as I could, pouring the boiling water into the teapot, 'we should think a bit more about our future.'

He finished checking the mail for any personal letters, but there were none. 'It's too soon,' he said.

'No, no, I'm not talking about children,' I smiled. 'I'm talking about making our home an investment. We should think about getting our own house while we're both working and we don't have any children.'

He stirred his cup. 'Mm. It's an idea.'

I thought of the cold, unwelcoming sitting room in the flat, his mother's cactus plant standing in the corner laughing at my attempts to kill it. No matter what I did, it survived. I hated cactus plants. They were so prickly, unattractive and unfulfilling.

'You know,' I continued earnestly, 'we're throwing our good money down the drain paying rent.' I swallowed quickly. 'We ought to get a place of our own, get a mortgage so that we own it in the end. It would make a good investment.'

'Yes, you may be right. I'll have a look around for us.' He put his cup firmly in his saucer and stood up. 'I need to go and check on my mother. I'll be back in an hour or so.' John left his tea unfinished. I sighed.

A few days later he bounded into the flat grinning and placed a file of papers on the table.

'Well, I've put a deposit down.'

'What, on a house? Where? What's it like? No chance for me to choose, then?' I looked at the file of papers.

'Well, you said it would be all right for me to choose. You're stuck in school all day.'

'I know. I know. It's all right,' I put a reassuring hand on his.

'Here you are.' He opened the file. 'There's a picture of it here. It's a semi-detached house in Sutton, right in the centre of my district and commutable for your teaching.'

'Just as well I trusted you, eh?' John was like a puppy wagging its tail vigorously. He was pleased and proud: mission accomplished. I'd known in my heart of hearts it had to be John who did the choosing. No matter how much I demanded to have what I wanted, we would never be happy unless John made the decisions. What did it matter? I could teach anywhere.

We moved into our semi-detached house in Sutton Drive in Sutton near Ely and soon assumed a role of domesticated bliss. We both went out to work, the housework hardly ever got done, but John made no complaints and I noticed he did not muck in either. We were happy in our new little home. There remained only one dark shadow over our lives — John's frequent visits to his mother.

One dull Saturday afternoon, I looked at the pile of ironing. I hated ironing, but it had to be done. John stood beside me.

'My mother used to iron my shirts perfectly,' he said, watching me heave the basket onto the sofa.

I was in no mood to be gentle. I pulled out the ironing board and made a big fuss of setting it up. I had no idea why he didn't offer to help, but I had other things to discuss.

'You know, John, you think you have full responsibility for your mother, don't you?' I grabbed the iron from the cupboard and plugged it in. 'You don't, you know.' I looked directly into his eyes. He looked perplexed.

I spat on my finger and touched the iron. It was hot enough. 'She's a grown woman. Besides, what about the rest of your family? Don't any of them see her? Why can't we ask them to help? Don't you have a grandmother and grandfather we should meet?' I picked up a shirt and put it on the ironing board.

'No, we're not going to see the rest of my family.' He stood stiffly watching me.

'Why not?' I swept the iron over his shirt, ignoring the extra crease I had made.

'We're not going to, and that's all there is to it. We have to be loyal to my mother,' John scowled.

'What about your aunts and uncles?'

'How do you know about them?'

'That's the whole point, I don't, but the picture I saw in your mother's house showed her surrounded by 4 other people. Besides, didn't you mention one of your uncles some time ago?'

'No, I didn't.'

I slammed the iron down. I was stunned. He *did* mention an uncle; I was sure of it, an Uncle Jim, so why deny his existence now? I moved his shirt over the ironing board ready to do the sleeves. The hiss of the iron left unattended on its stand interrupted the uncomfortable silence that filled the room.

I stuck my chin out. 'Listen, mate, whether you want it or not, I have a right to at least *meet* your other relatives, no matter how horrible they may be.' I grabbed the iron and swept it over his sleeve creating yet another crease. He'll just have to keep his jacket on, I thought.

The following Saturday, we were lying in bed. I could hear the birds outside, the village was sleeping and all was well. I listened. There was no phone call from his mother — yet. I leaned over him, placed my hand on my favourite spot on his slim chest and murmured, 'This would be a lovely day to go visiting.'

'Maybe,' John murmured.

'Why don't we visit one of your other relatives?'
He held me. 'No, I don't think that's a good idea.'
I extricated myself from his arms, slipped out of bed and wrapped my dressing gown around me firmly.

'I think it is a very good idea. We will visit one of your other relatives first and then I'll agree to go to your mother's afterwards. That's fair, isn't it? All right?' John frowned.

'Well?' I snapped.
His face paled. He got out of bed slowly. 'I'm not sure.'

'Listen, mate,' I hissed, 'I'm going to meet the rest of your family whether you like it or not. You phone around and find out whom we can see. If you don't do it today, I'll contact them behind your back. Do you want that?'

'No! No!' he said quickly. 'All right, all right. I'll phone grandmother. You won't like her. You'll regret it.'

I ignored him as I went into the bathroom to shower.

John drove slowly, his eyes set on the road ahead.

'But this is the way to Peterborough,' I snarled. 'We are *not* going to your mother's first. I simply won't get out of the car if we do.'

'Keep your hair on,' he snapped. 'We're going to see Grandmother. She lives in Peterborough too.'

I bit my lip. How could a mother and daughter live in the same city and not speak to each other? What a weird family this was. Maybe Granny would be the evil witch John had described. Well, no matter, I thought, wriggling into a more comfortable position in my seat, the one visit will suffice. At least we are meeting her!

'What happened to your grandfather?' I asked, keeping the tone casual.

'He had the good sense to leave her. She divorced him.' His pale face and tight lips made me decide not to ask any more questions about the grandfather.

I thought of our honeymoon and the couple from London who had mentioned a Mr Cox joining the gold rush in Bendigo, deserting his girlfriend? Could he be John's grandfather? Why the secrecy?

'Does your mother come and visit your grandmother sometimes?'

John gritted his teeth. 'No.'

'Why not?'

'It's none of you business. Grandmother is evil, you do not want to have anything to do with her or the others, believe me. If you knew what my mother has been through ...'

'Well, tell me then, so that I can understand.'

'No.'

'Listen, John,' I said, 'no matter what happened in the past, it is for us to form our own relationships with your other relatives and if they have done something dreadful and we find this out for ourselves, then and only then do we have reason to avoid them.'

I looked at the flat fields as the brick chimneys came into view. The scene felt particularly dull and uninspiring today.

Chapter 10

John's grandmother was a small round-faced woman who smiled as we entered her sitting room. She sat next to a warm coal fire. The house was dark but inviting, like an ordinary home rather than the cold pristine house of my mother-in-law.

She smiled. 'I am so glad to meet you,' she said.

'Me too,' I said.

She looked at John. 'You've grown into a handsome man, haven't you? How is Eunice?'

He fingered his tie. 'Fine,' he said coolly and held onto my arm. She leaned forward. 'I have not seen her for such a long time. I would love to see her. Her brothers and sisters come and see me,' she frowned.

John did not answer.

'Even Walter's brother visits occasionally. It was such a pity Eunice took our divorce so seriously. There was nothing I could do. Gerald took off with another woman, made it rich in Australia and gave her a large amount of his wealth. She has every reason to be happy. It is very strange,' she shook her head. Suddenly she looked up and looked directly at me. She looked me up and down. 'What size are you?' she asked. I gulped. This was a bit personal wasn't it?

'Er, about a twelve, I think.'

'I have a suit that you might like,' she said as she got slowly to her feet and stomped up the stairs.

There was a loud tap on her front door. I looked at John. He shrugged his shoulders.

'Get that will you?' Granny called from upstairs. John remained rooted to the spot. I sighed and went to the door and opened it. The man smiled. He was short, slim and dressed in a flashy suit. He reminded me of a much older and more flamboyant version of John. This man's brown hair was speckled with grey and his face was lined with years of experience. His light blue eyes twinkled with mischief like John's but they darted about the room a little more quickly and had a hint of wariness that I had never seen in John's. He held out his hand.

'I'm Matthew, Matthew Wilks. I've come to see Beatrice. Beatrice Cox?' He held out his hand.

'Oh yes, of course,' I shook his hand. 'I'm Sally, Sally Wilks. I married John.' I stepped back and let him in.

'Hello, John,' Matthew said cheerfully.

'Hello,' John mumbled. The clock on the mantelpiece ticked loudly as we stood in an uncomfortable silence, waiting for Granny.

'Won't be a moment,' she called from upstairs. Matthew coughed. 'How is Eunice these days?'

'She's fine,' John snapped, 'and she does not want to see you again.'

'John!' I stared at him. His nostrils flared and his eyes darkened.

'It's all right,' said Matthew holding out an open hand, 'I loved Eunice in my day but she married the better man. Isn't that right, John?'

John shrugged his shoulders. Matthew continued, 'I can understand why she doesn't want to see me.' He moved closer to John. 'It must be hard for you and your mother, John.'

John sniffed and stared at Matthew contemptuously.

'Perhaps it is better for Eunice and me if we don't meet,' Matthew stepped back a little. 'But I would love you and Sally to come ...'

'Sorry to keep you,' Granny interrupted loudly as she carefully stomped her way down the stairs. We watched until she had reached the bottom step safely. 'Ah, Matthew, it's lovely to see you.' She grinned. He stepped over and gave her a hug.

She turned to me. 'Here,' she pushed the garment into my hands, 'you take that home and see if it fits you. If it doesn't, give it to someone else.'

'Why, thank you,' I smiled. I felt brave now that Matthew was with us. 'Do you think Eunice will come to see you sometime?' I ventured. At last I managed to say John's mother's name out loud. At last she was a separate entity, not an extension of John.

'Ever since the divorce and your trouble, Matthew, she has not been near me. It is a pity. I would like to see her.' She looked wistfully out of the window.

'I know it has been awful for you, Beatrice.' Matthew moved nearer to her. 'I can assure you that you have done all that you possibly could. She can be very contrary sometimes. Sometimes you just can't help some people.'

What was horrible about these people? They seemed fine to me.

John stood up. 'Well, we must go.' He glared at me.

'But you've only just come,' said his grandmother, putting her hand out. 'Can't you stay a bit longer and have a cup of tea with Matthew and me?'

'No,' John snapped, and pulled me to my feet.

I smiled weakly at Matthew and Granny. 'I'm sorry our visit is so short. Thank you *so* much for the suit.'

John pulled me to the front door yelling 'Bye' as he opened it and we went outside. He closed the door firmly.

As I climbed into the car I asked, 'What was wrong with them? They both seemed fine. Why couldn't we stay and chat with Matthew?' I buckled my seatbelt.

John scraped the car into gear. 'What is *right* with them, you should ask. I wouldn't ask any more questions about them if I were you. Let sleeping dogs lie.'

We drove in an uncomfortable silence. My stomach constricted the closer we got to my mother-in-law's house. Eventually John swept the car into her drive. As he got out of the car, the window above was flung open. Mother-in-law scowled down at us.

'You're late! You said you were coming much earlier!'

'Yes, I know,' said John, 'we got held up. I'm sorry.'

'Don't you say sorry to me! You do just what you like and you're never sorry. I don't know why I agreed to your coming and bringing her anyway.' She waved a taut hand in my direction.

'Look, Mother,' John smiled, 'we have come all this way to see you, so why don't you let us in?'

'I've changed my mind. You can just turn around and go. I've had enough of you and your selfishness. I've been waiting here for ages. I boiled the kettle and now it's cold. I go to a lot of trouble to get ready for your visit and all you can do is turn up late and smile at me.

You've never been any good to me. I may as well go inside. I can look after myself. I don't need you!'

'But, Mother!' John cried.

'Huh!' she snarled. 'But Mother! What's that supposed to mean?' She slammed the window down with a thud. John looked up at the window. It remained firmly closed. The house stood cold and silent. He looked at the front door. Nothing happened. A car drove past the driveway. Some children chatted outside as they walked along the path but the front door remained firmly shut. John went to the front door and rang the bell. Nothing happened. He waited. He tried twice more. There was still no response. Eyes smarting, he turned and walked swiftly to the car. He started the engine and we drove home in an awkward silence.

The next day, when John had calmed down a little, I said, 'I would love to meet your other aunts and uncles, you know.'

John gritted his teeth. 'Would you!'

I stared straight into his troubled eyes.

'We might meet Uncle Tom another weekend perhaps.'

Who was Uncle Tom? What happened to Uncle Jim? Where did he fit into the picture? Maybe he had died already. I dared not ask and annoy John anymore; he was finding all this a bit much anyway. How could his mother behave in such a terrible way and yet have such a strong influence, so strong that John was unable to form relationships with the rest of his family? Something was seriously wrong and one day, one day, I would find out what it was.

Uncle Tom and Aunty Janice welcomed us with friendly smiles. Uncle Tom had the same shock of brown hair as John and his smile was a warmed-up version of Granny's but his complexion was more tanned and his cheekbones were more pronounced. Uncle Tom sat with John while I went to the kitchen to join Aunty Janice.

'It's lovely to meet you,' said Aunty Janice, a beautifully groomed woman much younger than John's uncle. 'Tom is a bit of an old stick but he's a good man.'

'Yes?' I watched as she balanced the tray ready to take into the sitting room. 'He can't stand children he says but he is good to my Elspeth. Elspeth is my daughter by my first marriage. After my first husband and I divorced, Tom took us on.' She lifted up the tray. 'He has been really good to us.'

'Here,' I said, rather too late, 'Let me help you.'

'No, no.' She opened the kitchen door. 'I'll be all right. You just follow me and help entertain Uncle Tom. He has been looking forward to seeing John and meeting you.'

As we entered the room Tom was saying, 'Your mother is a difficult woman. She did have an eye for the boys, though. That business about Matthew ...' He smiled at me, 'Well, I am pleased to meet you at last. So, a young Aussie, eh? Who'd have thought it?'

'It's amazing what you can pick up these days,' John grinned. 'Sally comes from Tasmania, you know.' I smiled quickly, noticing how John had interrupted so quickly. Was I going to get the whole story about his family? Obviously not on this visit. I decided not to intervene this time.

One Saturday evening, we were sitting watching TV.

'I hate the drive to school in Peterborough,' I sighed, simply speaking my thoughts aloud. 'The road by the forty-foot dyke is so dangerous and now that Winter is coming there will be all that ice to contend with. I'm still not sure what black ice looks like.'

'Well, get another job,' John said immediately. It seemed so simple to him.

'It's not that easy.' I got to my feet slowly, rummaged in the pile of newspapers on the desk and extricated the latest Cambridge Evening News. 'There are hardly any jobs to suit me. There is only one for a Head of Department.'

'Let me see.' John stood up quickly and came to peer over my shoulder. 'Fenton Village College. That's not too far. You should go for it.'

'You mean, just like that. I'm just an assistant and I've had only one job in this country. I'm not really ready for Head of Department am I?'

'Go on,' he insisted, 'live a little. What have you got to lose? After all, an idea that is not dangerous is unworthy of being called an idea at all. Go for it, girl. Send off an application tonight.'

'Well I suppose I could try.' I reached slowly for pen and paper to draft my application letter.

As I entered the stark waiting room, I saw four men perched upright on the row of seats. Obviously they were waiting to be interviewed too. That decided it. I had no chance. If I didn't know I would have to teach form 4R if

I went back to school early, I would have left immediately.

'Mrs Wilks?' My hands were shaking as I stumbled into the interview room. The row of earnest faces smiled weakly at me.

The room was spacious. A thin window stretched above the heads of the interviewers. They all looked old enough to be my father, except for the prim lady perched at the end.

'Why did you leave Tasmania?' the wrinkled governor of the school seated in the centre asked.

I did not bother to think too much. An inner voice reminded me I would not be getting the job, so it did not matter what I said.

'Oh, it was the Education Department,' I blurted out, my Australian accent sounding even more pronounced than usual. 'They would not pay a parent I had persuaded to teach violin so I upped and left.' I smiled. The governor sat back and looked at me squarely.

He asked some more common questions. I looked him straight in the eyes and answered candidly. The prim mistress asked me if I was married. She was obviously fishing to find out if I was pregnant. I evaded the issue. What right of hers was it to ask, or to try to ask, such personal questions?

'Have you any questions you would like to ask us?' the governor asked.

'What would the teaching load be?' I decided the longer I stayed there, the less likely it was that I would have to teach 4R today. Finally, I ran out of questions.

'Thank you,' the governor said, standing up and shepherding me out of the room. 'If you would wait with the others for a while, we will get back to you.'

I sat in the empty chair. I shrank into the empty chair. Being surrounded by a group of heavily suited experienced teachers did nothing for my confidence. I patted my leg with my hand nervously tapping out rhythms that were getting more and more frenetic as the time passed.

The door finally opened. I stopped tapping and the five of us stared with bated breath.

'Mrs Wilks, would you come in again please?' My inner voice decided that they were doing the refusals first. I was obviously bottom of the list.

'Please sit down.' I sat, forcing my face into a blank, noncommittal expression.

'We would like to offer you the job, if you will take it,' said the headmaster as he stood and came over to me.

I stared open-mouthed and only just stopped myself asking them if they had made a mistake. 'Er, I would love to!' I grinned, staggered to my feet and shook his hand.

I narrowly missed two cars on my euphoric drive home.

When John pulled up, took his jacket off and came into the house I threw myself at him.

'I've got it! I've got the job!'

'I said you could do it,' he grinned. 'That's great news.'

'I couldn't have done it without you.' We hugged.

John extricated himself. 'I must tell our friends. I'll ring Mother first.'

'You do that.' My voice was excited and pleased. There was no time for worrying about other things now. I'd done it!

'I'll go and do some preparation.' I rushed to my pile of school papers. It was going to be hard to be enthusiastic about my present school now, but I'd better do it all the same.

John hadn't heard. He had slipped upstairs to use the phone in his office.

.

Chapter 11

John had been working very hard in the last few months. I knew that he frequently visited his mother at the end of the day, but I decided to leave things as they were. It would do no good to complain and as long as it kept John happy, what was there to complain about? He no longer tried to force me to visit her every weekend; I could leave him to see to her needs as much as he could.

Then one Friday John was particularly late home. This time I knew where he had been. This time it was all right.

'It's the Norfolk Show!' he had announced the night before. He was smiling. 'I'll be on the Nelson and Hall stall. No doubt there will be a few beer tents to investigate with the lads too. I'll be back late tomorrow.'

'That's fine. Enjoy yourself. Bring me back a programme if you like.'

He was indeed late. He walked slowly into the house his face suntanned, his jacket covered in dust. We had an early night. I was glad of some extra sleep. We both climbed into bed and sleep overtook us. We were both very tired.

'Quick!' the voice was urgent. 'Quick, you've got to do something!'
I opened my eyes sharply. It was John sitting up and pointing to the corner of the room. I looked where he was pointing. Two blank walls greeted me.

'Look, there it is.' He pointed his finger excitedly, again and again.

'Where's what?' I asked, my words slurred as I tried to force myself awake.

'It's a bull, a huge bull,' he cried.

There was no bull.

'Oh, it's a bull,' I echoed. As if it was not enough that I was exhausted from a hard day's work and badly needed my sleep, I now had to be entertained by his dreams in the night.

'You must *do* something!' he shouted, his voice rising in agitation.

'Why me?'

'Quick, get hold of the bull. Take it out of the bedroom, *now*!'

'Anything for a quiet life,' I murmured as I slowly got out of bed, pretended to pull on the rope of a supposed bull in the corner of the room and lead it out of the bedroom.

'Right. He's out of the bedroom now. You can relax,' I said. I climbed back into bed pulled the covers towards me, turned away from him and shut my eyes. Please God no more dreams tonight.

The following week it was a sheep I was supposed to round up. I opened my eyes with a start. Oh no, he was at it again. What was it this time?

'Those sheep, they're going into the field. You've got to stop them.'

'Do I?' I snarled. I paused. I was supposed to help him get through this dream was I? But didn't I need my sleep too?

I snapped, 'You're dreaming. Turn over and go to sleep!' I did not care if I was doing the wrong thing. Anyway, why couldn't he do his own dirty work in his dreams? Why did I always have to be his slave?

One Thursday evening, John bounced into the dining room.

'I've been to see Sam.'

I was drooping over the pile of exercise books I had nearly finished marking. I was utterly sick and tired of trying to decipher the students' spidery scrawl. I had only three more to deal with. I was glad of the interruption. I paused, pen in hand.

John stood close to me, his eyes sparkling with energy. 'He's going to get his old Ford out. You and I can go as Bonnie and Clyde.'

I put another red mark through a student's work. What was he talking about? I thought back to last week's conversations. Oh yes, the Village Feast.

'Is it this Saturday?'

'Yes. We'll need to get up early to get ready. The parade for the Feast starts at 9 o'clock.'

Bang goes my lie in, I thought. What did I have in my wardrobe to wear? What did John have to wear for that matter?

'I'll wear my leather jacket. Sam's got a replica gun. That should do the trick.'

I tossed the exercise book on top of the pile and picked up the next one.

'Mm,' I murmured as I frowned at the scribble on the page.

'I'll just pop over the road to see how the Johnsons are doing.' The front door clicked.

I finished marking the books, shoved them in my briefcase and went upstairs to bed. John would come home eventually.

The morning of the Feast parade was dull. Billowing clouds hid the sun but they were mostly white and unlikely to shed their contents.

'Don't bring your coat,' John said as we left the house. 'It's not going to rain. I heard the forecast on Radio 4 when I got up to make the early morning cup of tea.'

I looked hesitantly at my raincoat, shrugged my shoulders and followed him as he walked swiftly towards the field. I puffed as I tried hard to keep up with him. Although short in stature, the long rapid stride he had developed from pacing farms on a daily basis was impossible for me to match.

'Wait!' I called to his leather-clad back. He did not hear me.

People, cars, tractors and trailers were gathering in the field. John disappeared in a kaleidoscope of colourful costumes, ribbons and balloons as the floats formed a ragged line.

I found John near the back of the queue talking earnestly to Sam, who was holding open the door of his black Ford. I could see Sam's buxom wife, Carol sitting in the passenger seat.

'I'll drive,' John said.

'No, it's OK,' Sam said swiftly, his smooth features interrupted with a deep frown. 'I'm the only one insured. I'll drive. You and Sally walk beside the car.'

John disappeared for a moment and returned with a bucket in his hands.

'Here, you take this.' He thrust it towards me. 'You can collect the money while I keep an eye on things ahead.' He dashed forward.

One after the other, the cars and tractors started their engines. The smell of petrol fumes mingled in the morning air with the busy excited chatter of the people. Sam turned the key and the Ford started immediately. The trailer in front of us jolted slightly, the huge pile of potatoes bouncing slightly as it edged forward. We were off!

'All right?' John spoke suddenly in my right ear. I jolted in surprise. I had not seen him coming. 'How do you like the gun? Not bad, eh?'

I smiled, still walking forward to keep pace with the car.

'Watch where you point it!'

'I'll hold up the onlookers, baby, you extract the cash.' He brandished the gun. 'Come on then, Eddy, cough up' He pointed the gun at a plump onlooker, who grinned as he put his hand in his pocket. 'And you too, lady.' A comely woman in a long pink dress delved into her little pink purse. My bucket rattled with coins.

John moved up and down the crowd of onlookers cajoling them to fill the bucket with their money. I wondered what I was going to do when the bucket got too heavy. I also wondered what we would do if the spots of rain that started falling became heavier and turned into a proper downpour. I brushed a spot of water from my nose. A little girl, her hair tightly pulled back in a ponytail, tentatively put her hand out and dropped a coin in my bucket. I smiled at her.

'Thank you, young lady, and some from your mum?' I waved the bucket under the nose of a tall thin woman with a close-fitting bonnet. Just as she was about to put in her contribution, there was an astonished cry from the onlookers. Open-mouthed they stared at the trailer in front of us. John's gun was on the ground next to an open sack of potatoes. A single potato rolled towards John's feet as he staggered towards the crowd, clutching his forehead. Blood oozed down his face.

I dropped the bucket and ran forward. 'John, what happened?' I cried.

'He tried to catch a sack of potatoes as it fell but bumped his head on the edge of the trailer.' Jack, a broad man, his tanned features creased with concern, took hold of John firmly by his shoulders. 'The doctor's clinic is still open. We'll take him there.' He held John steadily as he walked him away. 'We're lucky it's just up the road.'

My face drained of colour, my limbs quaking; I meekly followed the farmer who had his arms firmly round John's shoulders, half walking and half carrying him up the road. The float procession would have to do without Bonnie and Clyde for the moment. A voice spoke calmly in my ear.

'It's all right. I'll see to the bucket. You go on with your husband.'

Jack and John staggered on and up the path of the doctor's large brick residence. By now light rain was sprinkling on us as we struggled forward. I rushed in front of Jack and John to ring the bell. The door opened.

'M-my husband's had an accident,' I stuttered breathlessly.

'You'd better come in,' said the young, well-groomed receptionist as she opened the door wider, stepped back and failed to disguise the disgust on her face at the blood that splattered onto the carpet.

'His name?' she asked.

'Wilks, John Wilks,' I said quickly.

'I'll tell the doctor you are here.' She hurried further into the building.

Jack struggled with John into the waiting room and sat him down on the nearest empty chair.

'No relation to my old buddy Walter?'

'Yes, he was my father,' John said, his speech slurred.

'Ah,' Jack shook his head, 'such a shame he died so young. He was such a reputable man in the community. Although he and his older brother used to get into some scrapes when they were teenagers, I can tell you.' He paused. 'It was a terrible business about his brother though. It must have ruined your father. I'm sorry ol' chap,' Jack put his hand on John's shoulder. 'Still, you're in good hands now.' Jack straightened himself up and patted me on the arm. 'I'd better get back to my family.' He left before I could even mutter 'thank you' and much to my annoyance, before I could ask what he meant by 'the terrible business' about John's father's brother.'

John sat forward in his chair, the blood flowing profusely through his fingers, his features getting paler by the second. The receptionist was behind her desk.

'Have you got something to stem the flow of blood?' I shouted to her across the waiting room, making no effort to hide my irritation. Couldn't she see that he needed something to stop the bleeding? The receptionists blinked, her slim fingers hesitating. A moment later she came into the waiting room.

'This is all I could find,' she said meekly and with her arm stretched out she handed me a sanitary towel. She scuttled behind her desk. The intercom bleeped.

'John Wilks?' she called. I held John's arm and he stood up slowly, his hand clutching the sanitary towel over his forehead. Still holding onto John, I knocked on the surgery door.

'Come in,' called a deep voice, muffled by the thick door. 'Now what can be the matter ...?'He stopped mid sentence for it was painfully obvious what the matter was.

'Sit down, John. In the wars again, eh?' I grimaced. I did not like being reminded of all the other times we had been to the surgery because of John's talent for having accidents.

The doctor took a dressing from the shelf behind him, took away the sanitary towel, cast it into a bin and quickly applied the dressing. 'Can you hold onto this?' he asked John. John mumbled and held the dressing. The doctor pulled up a chair and sat opposite John.

'You're looking a bit pale. Any headache?'
John said, 'No.'

'Do you feel sick?'

'No.'

'Any trouble with your vision?'

'No.'

The doctor sat opposite John. 'Now let me look at the wound.' He lifted the dressing carefully and peeked at the wound before replacing the dressing straightaway.

'It looks fine. No stitches needed. I'll just clean it up and you can go on your way.'

The doctor got rid of the sanitary pad and taped a large fresh dressing to John's forehead. He walked to his desk and started writing.

John stood up. 'Great. We can get back to the Feast now.'

'Err ...' the doctor lifted his head quickly, 'I wouldn't do that if I were you. You should go home and lie down. Let me know if you have any headaches, sickness or problems with your vision.'

'Will you be going to the party after the Feast tonight?' John asked the doctor.

I pulled John's arm and said quickly, 'Thank you, doctor. We'll be off now.' I escorted John firmly out of the surgery. I steered him towards our house.

'It's okay,' he said, 'I'll just go and see what they're up to. I'll be back in a while.' He extricated himself from my arm and proudly wearing his badge of honour, a large white dressing in the middle of his forehead, he dashed towards the sounds that were coming from the field.

'On your head be it,' I grumbled as I walked home. I walked happily, noticing that the light rain had petered out and I could take my time walking along the narrow path. So his dad, Walter, was well known in the district. Surely it was something to be proud of, so why the secrecy? And what did Jack mean about his brother ruining him? One day I would discover the whole story.

Chapter 12

One Saturday afternoon the phone rang. John was upstairs at the time so answered it immediately.

'That was a phone call from Taru,' John called as he bounded down the stairs. I was sitting on the sofa with a pile of school papers trying to establish some semblance of order. I looked up.

'Taru?'

'Yes, she's the sister of my friend Karita. You know, the family in Finland I stayed with when I did my apprenticeship in agriculture.'

'Oh.' A sheet of paper fell to the floor. I bent down to pick it up and the rest of the pile spilled off my lap. I cursed under my breath.

'We're invited to go to her house for midsummer.'

'Midsummer?' I grumbled as I tried to gather the sheets together.

'The weekend after next. We're staying the weekend after next.' John stood watching me grovelling on the floor.

'It's in Cheshire?'

'I suppose so.' It was not as if I had anything better to do.

I felt the tensions of the previous week ease as we swept into the country. The flat Fens had given way to undulating green fields, quaint coppices and pockets of contented dairy cattle.

Taru and Howard's house was large and rambling, a monument to years of traditional dairy farming. .

'Come in, come in,' a round-faced but slim Taru greeted us, her strident voice coloured with a strong accent. Howard, her tall, thin, silent husband, stood beside her. She leaned her slim frame forward, gave John a big hug and stepped back to shake my hand. Howard shook our hands and stepped back, smiling shyly. A black cat and a line of kittens ran to Taru. She picked up the last kitten.

'You must take one of these kittens; they are ready to leave their mother now.' She put the kitten in my arms. I hugged it, stroking it until it purred loudly.

'I'd love a kitten, John.'

'All right, but we don't have a cat box to take it back in,' he said, as though we were accepting a bag of cabbages. 'Now, where are we staying?'

'We'll get you a box, don't worry. Now follow me.' Taru walked toward the open front door. 'I've put you two in the green room at the back. We'll have a sauna when you are ready. Howard will be seeing to the fire.'

'Sauna?' I asked meekly.

John opened the car boot. 'Yes, you know — a hot room where you get up a good sweat. It's very relaxing.' He took out our suitcases, closed the boot and walked towards the house. Taru and Howard by now had disappeared inside. I followed John through one dark corridor after another until we came to an open door at the back of the building. He put the cases down beside the huge double bed.

'She's left us some towelling robes. We'd better get ready.' John lifted his case up onto the bed, sprung it open and started hanging up his clothes in the spacious wardrobe. I copied him and my case was soon empty.

'What do you wear in the sauna?' I asked.

'Why, nothing, of course.' John started undoing his tie.

'Not even a swimsuit?' I looked longingly at mine before I closed the drawer.

'No. I think Taru said she has the silver birch twigs ready, didn't she?'

'Yes, I think she did say that,' I said absently. I was finding it difficult to come to terms with sitting in a sauna stark naked with Taru who was a very good friend of John's but a stranger to me. John was lucky, I moaned to myself. He had a lovely body. He was slim. I hated my extra rings of fat.

'They smell lovely after you beat each other with them.' John was already in his towelling robe.

'Pardon?'

'The silver birch twigs.'

'Oh.' I turned my back on John as I slipped out of my clothes and struggled into my robe.

Taru was already in the sauna when we got there.

'Come on you two. Get your robes off. It is so silly these people who are too shy to take off their clothes. It's perfectly natural after all.'
I crept in behind John.

'If you are not used to it, you'd better sit on the bottom bench.' Taru had a bunch of silver birch twigs in her hand and was beating her legs with them. 'Now tell me, John, how is your mother?'

'She's all right. She misses Dad a lot.'

'It was a difficult time for her when he died. His brother, your uncle Matthew had been in a lot of trouble before Walter and Eunice were married. I was so annoyed with him. We had shares in his company, you know. He *was* good at his business and he sold us a good car, but we had no idea what he'd been doing.'

'Mm,' John murmured. 'We're going to my father's grave next week. It will be mother and father's wedding anniversary.'

For a brief moment I hung onto the words 'Uncle Matthew'. So, he sold cars and had been in a lot of trouble. There was little sign of this when I met him at John's grandmother's house. I felt too lazy to wonder why Taru was annoyed with him. Taru's and John's voices faded as I sat huddled on the bottom bench succumbing to the somnambulant effect of the hot surroundings. The smell of warm timber and the scent of silver birch were very soothing. I stretched out.

'Sally! Sally!' Taru's voice echoed in the back of my mind. I opened my eyes with a start.

'Ah, you're awake,' she smiled. 'Would you like a cold shower or are you going for a swim in the lake with John and me?

I tried to focus. What can you say when you don't want either?

'A shower,' I said, praying that there would be a hot tap as well as the cold.

There was no hot tap. I had the quickest shower I can ever remember, dressed hurriedly and went outside to watch John and Taru swim in the lake. The water stretched as far as I could see. Two little heads were just visible moving towards a tiny island in the centre of the water. I watched as the heads turned and started moving in my direction. Taru's voice wafted in and out of my hearing as she continued to chatter with John. I averted my eyes as two naked bodies finally climbed out onto the grassy verge.

'That was invigorating,' John grinned, reaching for his towelling robe. 'You should try it.'

'I might go for a little swim next time,' I lied.
Taru was in her robe rubbing her hair with a towel. 'After you're dressed, we'll go and see how Howard is getting on with the fire.'

By sunset, the field next to the house was buzzing with the excited chatter of neighbours gathered round a huge pile of off-cuts, logs and debris from the farm. Howard was about to light the fire.

'Would you like to help me pass round the Sima? Taru asked.'

'Sima?' I queried.

'Yes, it's a drink we make when we have celebrations. It is very healthy. I'll give you the recipe later.'

We went into the kitchen where a huge bucket stood on the table. Taru ladled some of the fizzy fruit drink into glasses on a tray. I carried the tray out to the crowds and started distributing drinks.

John helped Howard add more logs to the fire and chatted to the people, their faces glowing in the firelight as sparks floated high into the darkening sky. There was no sign of the cats.

'Now for a song.' Taru grabbed the hands of people either side of her. 'Come on, link arms.' Her local friends, unaccustomed to Taru's Finnish traditions, tentatively linked arms and made a circle round the fire.

Taru sang lustily in her native tongue. No one knew the songs but hummed along with her as best as they could. Taru's strident tones filled the night air. Crackles from the fire interspersed her singing and the smell of burning logs grew stronger.

'John!' Howard shouted. 'No!' His voice was urgent. John had emerged from the farm outhouse where the debris for the fire had been stored. He was clutching a petrol can. He stood poised ready to toss it into the flames. The can rose high in the air.

'Get back! Get back!' Howard bellowed. The singers stopped mid-song. Open-mouthed they stumbled back away from the fire. A tremendous boom and flash of fire emanated from the bonfire. The onlookers' open-mouthed faces lit up as the blast ripped into the night air. They screamed. Debris from the fires lay scattered across the field, the smoke from it screening their astonished faces. Only the crackling of the fire remnants could be heard as the stunned onlookers stared at the blackened debris.

'My skirt!' a plump woman yelled. A thin line of smoke rose from the hem of her voluminous orange dress.

'I'll get it.' A wiry man in dungarees tossed his drink over the smouldering area on the skirt.

'You'd better go inside and change. I have a robe you can wear.' Taru put her arm round the sobbing woman. 'Is everyone else all right?'

The now-thinning crowd mumbled positively. As Taru escorted the woman into the house, Howard shook hands with his neighbours as they left quickly, one after the other. Finally Taru, John, Howard and I stood alone watching the last car make its hasty exit out of the drive way.

'Why did you do it?' I shouted at John. 'What on earth possessed you?'

'No harm done.' He grinned. 'It was only an old can that needed to be got rid of. I don't know what all the fuss is about.'

I looked at him closely. It was then that I began to question whether my lovely husband, my rock, my man, *was* the knight in shining armour I thought I had married. Did he not see the danger? Was I making a lot of fuss over nothing?

Howard and Taru murmured together looking at John. They, too, had their concerns.

After a restless night, we had an early breakfast and were soon packed ready to leave.

'We promised you a cat,' Taru said hesitantly, 'I think it should be your cat, Sally. Howard, go and get the box and the kitten will you?' Howard turned and went back towards the farmhouse. Taru smiled.

'What are you going to call the kitten?'

'I don't know.'

'As he is from good Finnish stock, and he is black, I think you should call him "Musta". It means "black" in Finnish.'

'Yes, Musta, we will call him Musta. All right, John?'

John nodded as he took the wriggling box Howard handed him and put it on the back seat of the car. As we drove out of the yard, I turned to wave to Taru and Howard. They had their arms linked and were waving back, but even at this distance the concern on their faces was clearly apparent. I looked back at the box on the car seat. It was quiet.

Chapter 13

One Saturday, many months later, after I had had a glorious uninterrupted full night's sleep, John was digging in the garden. He came into the house and found me in the kitchen.

'Come with me.' He tugged my arm. I was in the middle of peeling vegetables. I put the knife down and followed him down to the bottom of the garden.

'Look what has grown here.' It was a type of lily, charming, natural, and wild.

'It's lovely. What's it called?'

'It's called "Lords and Ladies". It's a woodland plant from the Araceae family. It's also called "Cuckoo Pint".' He bent down to admire the lily. Musta, now nearly fully grown, came up behind him and wrapped his body around his legs. John ignored the cat and continued, 'The male and female flowers are at the bottom of that poker-like protuberance and little hairs capture insects that get dusted with pollen as they struggle to escape. Later it will produce large red berries that are highly poisonous, but it is a beauty isn't it?'

I picked Musta up and held him until he wriggled. I put him down. I looked at John. He was teaching me more and more about this new country of mine. He was like an encyclopaedia; he knew facts, figures, history, quotations and jokes. I could listen to him for hours. In spite of my misgivings after our visit to Taru's I thought what a wonderful father he would make. After all, no one is perfect. No one had been hurt at the bonfire. He had just been over-enthusiastic, and what was wrong with enthusiasm?

But no babies arrived. We had been trying for a year. I was grateful for having a small bundle of fur to talk to and hug in moments when I pined for a baby. It did not seem natural not to have one.

'I agree you should have been successful by now.' The doctor scribbled onto his pad. 'I will send you both for tests.'

'Unto the breach I go,' John called as he opened his car door. 'As Oscar Wilde said, "You know there are only two tragedies in life: one is not getting what one wants, and the other is getting it."' He climbed into the front seat of his white Ford Escort and sped off to the hospital to have his tests.

I went for my tests too.

'You'll never guess.' John grinned from ear to ear waving the letter he had just received from the hospital: 'I'm not just fertile, I'm *super* fertile. How about that!'

I was never going to live it down. I was too, but nowhere near 'super fertile'. Our inability to conceive was a puzzle. In the back of my mind I wondered if John's bouts of bad mood and his inability to sympathize with my hurt feelings when he spent so much time with his mother had anything to do with it. The tension I felt whenever I had to meet his mother did not help. When we actually stayed at her place for one night, I noticed John did not dare come near me. But conceiving is a physical thing, not psychological, I told myself. Well, that was what I believed at the time.

One night when we were dining with our old friend Babs, John said, 'My wife is studying for another degree.' He could not help glowing with pride. 'She's going away for the week, on a compulsory week's study.'

'You'll have to come over to me for a meal or two while she's away.' Babs piled John's plate with potatoes. John smiled. He was going to be fine while I was away.

The course was at Sussex University. I stood at the notice board and worked out what I would be doing for the week.

'Is this your first summer course?' A man the same height and build as one of my previous boyfriends was reading the board too. I flushed. My heart had been broken dramatically by that ex-boyfriend and I could not help my heart stirring yet again, even though I was now married, definitely married. I was determined not to be tempted again by any charming look-alike.

'Yes. It looks an interesting programme.' I glanced at the social programme. 'Plenty of time to let our hair down too. I think I'm going to enjoy it.'

'Me too. Perhaps I'll see you around ...' He winked and walked away. His steady gait reminded me of ... I shook my head. I would have none of it.

'Well, hello again.' He stood next to me in the lecture room. We were attending the same classes.

'Dennis,' he said, shaking my hand. 'Dennis Parker.' His handshake was strong, warm and inviting.

'Sally,' I blushed, 'Sally Wilks.' We sat down next to each other. The electricity between us was undeniable. We sat upright in our chairs, ignoring the tension we felt, and conversed inanely before the lecturer entered the classroom. No matter what we did, which different events we tried to attend, we could not help gravitating towards each other. I now knew that when people said, 'It just happened', they were not lying. It could easily 'just happen' between us.

'I'm a married woman,' I blurted as we sat close to each other at one of the social events.

'I am too.' He gripped his thighs firmly. 'Well, a married man that is.'

'There's nothing for it,' I moaned, 'we'll have to sit in public the whole time we're together.' He did not need an explanation. We went to every lecture, every afternoon event and every public evening event we could, staying up until the very last moment so that we would be tired and ready for sleep — nothing more. The hormones were raging.

'I'd like to keep in touch.' Dennis held my arms. I longed to fall into his, but I was determined to remain strong.

'Me too,' I knew there was not much point in lying, 'But we shouldn't, really we shouldn't.'

'I'll look out for you at the next meeting in Cambridge.'

'Go,' I said, giving him a gentle push, 'get onto your train. I'll catch mine in a few minutes.' I pulled out a hanky, wiped away the tears that were falling down my cheeks, blew my nose and walked purposefully towards my train.

I leaned back on my seat. I closed my eyes. I could feel Dennis's presence close to me. If we hadn't been married ... I shook my head. The week was over and that was that. I must put him out of my mind.

I finally arrived home. John opened the door quickly before I had time to put my key in the lock. I hugged him hard and he pulled me inside, leaving my case in the doorway. 'I have something special for you.' He pulled two tickets out of his pocket. 'I've bought two tickets for us to see the Proms.'

I checked the tickets. There were only two this time. His mother would not be coming. I grinned.

'Lovely, I'm really looking forward to it. I never managed to go to one when I lived in London. This is wonderful, John.' I paused. I must get my case. I turned and fetched it, closing the front door behind me. I had to tell him sometime. I could not keep my feelings a secret. I would blurt it out sometime, so this was probably the best time, when he was in a good mood. He looked at me, fresh, open and ready.

'I think I should tell you something.' I looked into his pale eyes. He raised his eyebrows.

'What?'

'N-nothing happened,' I stuttered. 'Nothing happened,' I repeated earnestly, 'at the course, I mean, but I think we need to talk.'

He looked confused. I pulled him over to the sofa and sat down. He sat down next to me. I turned to him. There was only one way to say it and that was to say it immediately and directly.

'I nearly had an affair while I was on the course.' His face paled. My pulse increased as I forced myself to continue. 'But I didn't. John, really, I didn't.'

He froze.

I continued, 'I think our marriage is far too important. All right?'

His body stiffened.

'John? Please,' I pleaded, 'we should talk ...'

'No!' His face clouded. He clenched his teeth. He clasped me to him as if to expunge any feelings I may have developed for anyone else. Tears gathered in my eyes.

'Don't cry.' His voice was harsh. 'I can't stand you crying. I've seen enough crocodile tears in my time. It's no good you trying.'

We did not talk that night.

The Albert Hall was golden, the audience excited and colourful. This should have been one of the best moments of my life. I looked down at the orchestra. The conductor raised his baton and the music started. My raw emotions were roused even further. I watched the violins sweeping their bows across the strings through a thin veil of tears. John was unmoved, enjoying a night at one of his country's finest events.

Within a month I was pregnant. I was sure the hormonal boost I had been given by Dennis had done the trick, but I could not share that with John!

'I'm going to be a father!' John made sure the whole village knew within a few hours. He came home late many nights after celebrating his new status with his colleagues.

I smiled. He was indeed going to be a father and he would make a good one, I was sure of it.

'I'm going to a conference today. A colleague is picking me up. Some of my colleagues are coming here needing a lift too. You can drive them to Cambridge, can't you?' John put his coat on, gave me a peck on the cheek and opened the front door.

'What if I don't want to be a taxi for your colleagues?' I blurted.

'Oh, you'll be all right.' He patted me on my bottom, walked smartly to the waiting car outside, climbed in gave me a grin and a wave and the car left. I watched as it turned the corner and disappeared.

I opened our garage. I walked to the front of the car, got into the driver's seat, stretched over my bulge, put the keys in the ignition and started the car. Straining to turn my body to see out of the back window, I carefully backed the car out onto the driveway. It was still running when I walked past the exhaust pipe to close the garage door. I was suddenly overwhelmed with a desire to vomit. I stood aside from the fumes and waited. The feeling passed. I muttered to myself. Yes, I was indeed very pregnant and very sensitive but why didn't John notice? Where was my knight in shining armour, the one I thought would look after me, especially now? I sighed and gave the arriving colleagues a large false grin.

The next day I went for my check-up at the GP's.

'The baby is sitting in an odd position.' The kindly doctor smoothed her hands over my bump again. 'Just one moment.' She left the room. I was alone, left like a stranded seal, a large lump on the bed. I felt my bump. Was that an arm or a leg? Maybe it was two legs! I gasped. The GP finally re-entered the room with another doctor, saying to him, 'What do you think?'

He felt the bump and murmured softly. 'Maybe you're right. I'm not sure either.'

'What's wrong?' I asked, unable to conceal the agitation in my voice.

'No, no. There's nothing wrong. Do you have twins in your family?'

'Well, my grandfather was a twin. I'm not sure about John's family. Why?'

'Well, it's just that I think you may have twins.'

I paused for a moment. The news sank in. Wow! I clambered off the bed, dressed as quickly as I could and went to find John. He was standing at the kitchen sink, starting to make a cup of tea.

'The doctor thinks it's twins,' I blurted. John stopped what he was doing.

'Here', he said, steering me firmly to a seat in the dining room. 'You'd better sit down.'

'I'm *fine* but you look a bit pale. Don't you think *you* should sit down too?' John sat and we contemplated a very different kind of future.

Chapter 14

My bump and I continued to live as though circumstances had not changed.

'Maybe it is only one, after all,' the doctor commented as she began her inspection of the bump. 'Here are the two arms and the two legs. Yes, it is only one.'

'Oh,' I tried to hide the disappointment in my voice.

The bump grew and grew, sitting close to my chest. Feelings of nausea swept over me at a whim.

Babs and I were in the dining room. I had cooked us some chops and vegetables. Babs would eat anything, she said, as long as she didn't have to be at home before seven so she didn't have to answer all those phone calls one of her patients kept making.

'Although Allen can deal with them, I'd hate him to have to do it all night,' she said. She lowered her voice. 'While John's not here, you know Allen found out something about the Wilks family, don't you?'

'Oh?' I said, leaving the food on the stove so that it did not get too cold.

'Yes, we were clearing the loft of some old papers and he found a file marked Matthew Wilks.'

'Really?' my pulse thudded.

The phone rang. I muttered as I realized John was still outside so I had to answer it on the extension downstairs.

'Hello?' I blurted, annoyed with the interruption.

115

'Is John there, please?' I gulped. It was my mother-in-law. 'I'll get him!' I snapped and rushed to the backdoor. Really, her timing was incredible. I was dying to know what Babs had found out.

'John?' I called hurriedly. There was no reply, but I could see him working in the bottom of the garden. 'John?' I yelled. 'Your mother's calling?' He did not hear me. I had had enough. I went straight back to the phone and picked up the receiver.

'I'm sorry; he's at the bottom of the garden and can't hear me. We're about to have dinner, so I'll get him to call you back later, All right?' I said hurriedly. The sigh at the other end of the phone made it clear that it was not all right. I put the phone down before anything further could be said.

'You were saying?' I quickly sat down opposite Babs.

'I say,' Babs stood up and went to the stove, 'any chance of having this lovely dinner before it burns?'

'Oh, sorry, of course.' I stood up and joined her. My stomach churned with the smell of the food. 'I'd better dish up now.'

'I'll call John, shall I?' Babs said. I dished out the food onto the plates as quickly as I could. I needed to eat very soon if I was not going to be sick.

'Dinner!' Babs shouted. The whole neighbourhood now knew we were having dinner but at least John would have heard it. .

'Okay' John replied, but he continued tying the runner bean plants to stakes he had put into the garden.

I sat at the table and waited, my stomach gearing up for action. Babs sat down with me.

'A bit of a slow coach, isn't he?' she laughed. Nothing fazed her. I grimaced at her.

The light reflected on his shirt as he went into the back of the garage. He did not come into the house. His shirt lit up again as he returned to the garden.

'Really!' I stood up and leaned out the back door 'John!' I screeched and came back in and sat down.

'Go for it, girl!' said Babs.

I screwed up my face. I felt faint, consumed with the strong feeling of nausea. I sat down heavily, lowering my head only to lift it up swiftly when the smell of the food hit me again.

John called: 'I'll be there in a minute.' We could hear him clanging about in the back of the garage. This was too much.

'Sorry, Babs,' I muttered hurriedly, 'you carry on.' I dashed upstairs to the bathroom and just made it to the toilet bowl. Oh, how I hated vomiting. When I finally returned to the dining table still clutching a wet cloth John was seated at the table. I sat down and barked:

'Look, John, when I call you to dinner, you have to come straight away. You seem to have forgotten that I'm pregnant. If I don't eat straight away, I vomit. Okay?' I pushed my bump out to emphasize my point.

Babs smiled. 'Quite right too, you listen to your woman, John, she is a delicate little thing.'

I gave her a gentle punch on her arm. Why did she have to make a joke out of everything? I was serious.

He looked blank, as though he were being harangued by a demented stranger and her weird friend.

'Okay,' I said, 'I think in future, if you don't come to the table straightaway, I'll start without you.'

He shrugged. 'We're going to get a good crop of runner beans this year. Maybe we'll have enough for me to give some to my mother?'

'Ah, now there's an idea,' Babs grinned.

'Maybe not,' I mumbled into my food that was now cold.

It seemed hours before John went upstairs and Babs and I were left alone to clear up the dinner plates and finish our previous conversation.

'So,' I said stacking the plates. 'What *did* you find out about the Wilks family?'

'Allen's colleague had to represent Matthew Wilks in court. There was a scandal about him and his girlfriend.'

'I think Matthew Wilks is John's uncle — his father's brother. He sold cars. What had he been up to?' I put the plates into the sink and ran the tap.

'He'd been caught stealing from his company. The company collapsed. He reckoned he hadn't done anything wrong. He said his girlfriend had done it, but everyone knew he was lying, the evidence was damning. He would never reveal who his girlfriend was and ended up in jail for a while, poor chap.'

'Oh my goodness!' I gulped, just managing to turn the tap off before the sink overflowed.

'I wouldn't worry too much about it, Sally; it doesn't mean John's going to do the same.' She patted my shoulder. 'I'd just keep hold of the purse strings if I were you, just in case.' I turned around.

She smiled. 'Then you'll still be able to buy that bottle of champers we're going to share one day.' Her eyes twinkled.

I turned back to the sink. How could she make a joke of it! No wonder John and his mother would not talk about Matthew Wilks. I pursed my lips. How dare his mother question *my* background!

Every day for the next three days, John was late back from work. He offered no excuse. He was preoccupied. If it had only been one or two days, he would have been to his mother's, but now it was becoming very regular, too regular, surely, to be at his mother's every time. Even she must need a break from him sometimes. I scrutinized his shirt collars, looked at the contents of his jacket and trouser pockets before having them cleaned. It was very unlikely he was having an affair.

One day I could stand it no longer. He pulled up in the drive, swung open the car door and climbed out. Taking hold of his brief case he walked slowly to the door.

'Where have you been?' I tried to keep my voice light. 'You've been late every day this week.'

'Work,' he snapped.

I went into the kitchen and put the kettle on.

'Cup of tea?'

'No, I've already had some.'

'Was it with one of your clients?'

'No.'

I waited.

His lips curled in anger: 'Well if you must know, I've been having tea with my mother.'

'What *every* day?'

'So, what of it?'

'What about all the clients you are supposed to see?'

'I won't tell you when I see Mother next time. Then you won't make such a fuss about it.'

I pushed out my bump. 'You should be near home as much as possible. You have other responsibilities now. You need to be near me, just in case.'

'I've got work to do.' He turned towards the stairs.

'Before you go, tell me, why didn't you tell me about your uncle, Matthew Wilks?

'It's none of your business. Just keep out of it if you know what's best for you!' he snarled, and stormed up the stairs to his office.

I watched as he disappeared at the top of the stairs. I listened but I did not hear the click of the telephone.

I bent down and picked up Musta, who was curling round my leg. I stroked him. He purred. I buried my face in his warm fur. I vowed that the next time I was in town I would go to the library and search old newspapers. I was determined to find out the whole story about Matthew Wilks. Perhaps he was innocent as he claimed, although Babs seemed quite sure he wasn't, but mistakes have been made. I was certain about one thing — John would not talk about him anymore.

The next day John stayed in his office till late in the morning. I paced the sitting room floor eager to dash to the library after he had gone. The traffic outside was noisy. A car screeched its brakes. At last I heard the thump of John's files upstairs. He was packing, ready to go out. The doorbell rang. I opened the door.

'Do you own a black cat?'

'Yes we do and he's missing! Why?'

'There has been an accident.'

'Musta?' A cold shiver shot down my spine. 'Musta?' I called. I remembered seeing him last night, but this morning? He had not turned up for breakfast this morning.

'Excuse me for a moment please,' I said, 'While I look for our cat. Musta!' I called loudly through the house; I ran to the back door and shouted. But no Musta came. I rushed to the front door again.

By now John had heard the commotion and had joined me. We both stared at the slim lady in front of us, her expression fixed.

'I'm very sorry to have to tell you, but a black cat has been killed on the road. I wondered if it was yours. I do hope I'm wrong about this.'

'Where?'

'Around the back of your house. I'll show you.'

John and I, hand in hand, followed the lady, who led us around the corner and along the path that ran at the back of our house. There, lying flat and absolutely still, was our beautiful Musta.

'Oh, Musta,' I cried as I knelt down to him.

John put his hand on my shoulder. 'I'll pick him up and bury him in our garden.' Without another word spoken, he picked Musta up and slowly and carefully carried him home. I watched as he dug a hole next to the Lords and Ladies at the bottom of the garden and fashioned a tiny cross. We stood arm in arm for a while, remembering our little friend.

As we stood together, I knew that deep down inside the John I had married there was indeed compassion and understanding. He and I were feeling the same deep sense of mourning. Things would be all right. I no longer felt a great urgency to find out about his family. It was John I had married and only John I wanted. His family could wait.

After two more months, I was half way through my meal one night when John joined me at the table.

'Only a five weeks to go,' I said, sitting down heavily after producing his meal from the oven. He half smiled.

'I'll keep the car topped up with petrol.' He played with the food on his plate.

'Are you going to come with me to the concert in the village hall tomorrow night?'

'I'd like to, but I have a lot of paperwork to catch up on.' He took a mouthful of mashed potato.' He swallowed hard. 'Tonight I have a meeting about the village Feast. I need to get ready for it. Sorry, but I'm not hungry,' he said pushing the food to the side.

'The choir will be here to practise tonight,' I said.

'I'm going upstairs to get the paperwork ready for the meeting. Enjoy the cats' chorus.' He grinned and left the table.

'Cats' chorus?' I called after him. 'I'll have you know we are now famous after the press has put our picture in the paper.'

'That's because most of you are pregnant,' he called from the top of the stairs. 'No, I was only kidding. I do like to hear you all sing.' I heard his footsteps cross the landing to his office.

The next night I went to the concert alone. I squeezed my large body into one of the chairs at the back of the hall.

'How's the baby?' Agnes, a member of the choir and local health visitor, asked.

'Fine.' I forced a smile. 'I can't wait for it to come.' I stayed in my chair.

'Actually,' she leaned forward, lowering her voice, 'I'm so glad you came. I wonder if you could help me?' I raised an eyebrow. I wasn't exactly in any kind of fit state to do anything constructive.

'It's just that my mother is here with me.' Agnes jerked her head in the direction of the seats to the right. A kindly old woman, her wispy grey hair brushed neatly to the side, smiled weakly in our direction. 'I need to stay on to help clear up. Could you see my mother home at the end of the concert?'

'Er —'

'You'd be doing me a tremendous favour.'

'What if I start producing?' I patted my bump.

'Oh, you'll be all right.' She punched my arm affectionately.

Said mother was escorted home. I walked the rest of the journey alone to my own house, muttering under my breath. I changed lethargically, and pulled my large frame into bed next to John. He murmured in his sleep. I was exhausted and yet anxious, irritated and restless. I lay on my back, wishing the baby would come soon, dozing and dreaming of motherhood.

Then, suddenly, I felt wet. I was leaking.

Chapter 15

I dashed as fast as my heavy body could go and sat on the toilet. Water poured out. Surely it wasn't time? I hadn't felt any contractions. Anyway it had stopped just as suddenly as it started. I paced the landing. I went into our bedroom.

'John?' I prodded John's back. He stirred a little and murmured. 'What should I do? It's midnight and I'm not sure but I think something is happening.' He murmured more but was clearly not awake to really focus on what I was saying.

'I think I'll ring Agnes. They're probably still awake.' I still felt peeved that I had been neglected by so many in spite of my special condition. I picked up the phone and dialled.

'Hello,' a tired voice said unenthusiastically.

'It's Sally here.'

'Oh, yes, thank you for bringing Mother home.'

'Oh, no trouble. I hope you don't mind my ringing you at this ghastly hour, but something's happened. I think my waters have broken but it's weeks before the baby is due and I haven't felt any contractions or anything. What should I do?'

'When did it happen?'

'A few minutes ago.'

'Are you having any contractions now?'

'No.'

Agnes paused.

'I think you'd better be on the safe side. Ring the hospital and see what they say.'

Fumbling with the phone directory, I found the number of the ward and dialled.

'Hello, Maternity Ward,' a friendly voice said quickly.

'Hello. This is Sally Wilks. My baby is not due for 5 weeks but I think my waters have broken. The health visitor says I ought to ring you.'

'You did the right thing. I think you should come in. Have you transport?'

I looked at my sleeping husband.

'Yes, my husband can bring me in.'

'If you have any problems just dial this number again.'

'Thank you.' I dropped the receiver and it rattled in its cradle.

'John, John, wake up!' I staggered to the bathroom. I had not even got a sponge bag or nightdress sorted. It was far too early. I grabbed what I could and shoved them in a bag.

'John, John!' I yelled. This time I shoved him in the back until he finally moved a little and muttered.

'What?' his voice was drugged with sleep. 'Surely not at this hour. What time is it anyway?' His voice trailed away as he curled up and went to sleep again.

'No, John, don't go to sleep!' I pushed him again. 'It's the baby. The health visitor says we should go to the hospital NOW!'

'Oh, all right then.' He stretched slowly, opened his eyes a little and stared. He fumbled into some clothes and we went to the car.

The night was clear and cold. There were no other cars on the road. John drove at a steady pace, still trying to focus his eyes from his strong desire for sleep. Eventually we arrived at the hospital car park. He pulled into one of the parking bays and we walked together to the maternity ward. I felt no contractions so we were not in a hurry.

'It'll be all right,' I reassured him. 'It will be a false warning. Many people have one of those and have to go home again.' He nodded, still too tired to comment.

I felt intimidated as we walked along the wide brilliantly lit corridor. We were shepherded into a room near the entrance to the ward. I climbed onto the trolley and the doctor investigated the bump. I felt an enormous contraction. I had never felt anything like it before. It was horrible. It was one of the most ghastly deep-seated pains I had ever felt. What happened to the dream I had of feeling that nature and I would be as one, that I would have an involuntary urge to push the baby out into the world and nature would be with me? The moment of severe pain I felt was alien; there was nothing natural, about it.

'I can feel the placenta. The baby is in distress. We will have to do an emergency caesarean,' the doctor said quickly. 'Mr Wilks, you will have to leave the room.'

'Mrs Wilks, sign this paper please so that we can operate.' A sheet of paper was placed on my bump. I signed with my right hand, while my left hand was being strapped and a needle put into it. I was immobilized. I felt a searing pain as the knife sliced and dug into the bottom of my stomach. The pain was unbearable. I could not move or cry out. Darkness overwhelmed me.

'Ooh, how I hurt.' I awoke to an unbearable throbbing in my stomach. I had never felt so sore before. I dared not move for each tiny movement stirred the wound that was causing the excruciating pain.

'You have a lovely baby daughter.' The nurse placed a small bundle onto my arm. The baby was so small, small enough to fit between my wrist and my elbow. She had red hair and spindly legs.

'Are you sure this is mine?' I asked.

'Yes, of course she is,' the nurse said. 'She is a very strong baby. Even though she is only three pounds she does not need to go into an incubator.'

I tried to show interest but remained glued in a prone position. It was just too painful to move.

'I was the first to see her,' John said standing next to my bed, grinning. 'They said as soon as they got her out that she had red hair and that we would have to watch her temper. What shall we call her?'

'I've always liked the name Penny.' I tried to smile, but I could not, the pain was overwhelming. 'I have two really good friends and they are called Penny.' I wished I could sit up normally and hold the baby properly, but I couldn't. 'Would you like to hold her?' I asked John. 'Make sure you hold her head,' I murmured and I let John take the baby. He grinned as he had never grinned before. 'Yes, Penny, we will call her Penny.' He grinned at the tiny little face that dozed in his arms. 'I'll take her to show her to the friends who are waiting outside the ward.'

The nurse stepped forward.

'I'll be back in a minute.' John held his daughter in front of him, his face contorted with emotion. The nurse followed him closely behind. I remained frozen, willing the pain to go away.

The nightmare began.

'She seems to want a feed every hour,' I said as Sarah sat next to me. I was so thankful Sarah, seasoned mother of three, had come to see me.

'Are you demand feeding?' her confident smile eased my anxiety.

'Yes, I suppose I am. She is so small and we have to keep waking her up by tickling her toes because she is not big enough yet to feed naturally.'

'Mm,' Sarah patted Penny's shawl sympathetically.

'Mrs Wilks, there was a phone call for you,' the nurse said as she plonked a vase of Sarah's flowers on my bedside table. 'It was your mother-in-law wanting to know what she should bring when she comes. Did you want flowers or fruit?'

'Mother-in-law!' I sat up and screeched in pain. I had forgotten how much it hurt to move. I lay down again, holding my stomach. 'Not Mother-in-law, please. I have enough to worry about without having to deal with her.'

'It's all right, it's all right.' Sarah patted my bed and nodded to the nurse. 'I'll contact her.' She leaned closer to me. 'We'll do a rota of visitors so that you do not have to see her at the moment.'

'Will you? Oh, thank you!' I lay back a little and relaxed as much as I could. Penny wriggled in the trolley next to us.

The nurse took hold of the trolley. 'I'll bring her back for the next feed, all right?'

'Thank you. Thank you, Sarah' I drifted off the sleep. I did not see Sarah go.

I woke with a start. 'What are you going to do about contraception?' a strong voice interrupted my doze. Contraception? I thought. That's the last thing on my mind at the moment! The painful scar across my tummy smarted.

A nurse stood at the side of my bed. 'You know,' she said in clipped officious tones,' 'you are particularly fertile now you have just had a baby?' I didn't, but I hardly thought it would matter in my case. I would be in no fit state to do any of that kind of thing for a long time. I put it to the back of my mind.

'It'll be all right,' I sighed. Penny was asleep in a trolley next to me. I turned over again to sleep while I could.

The baby stirred. My body ached with exhaustion. Not another feed! I picked up Penny.

'Hello,' John's cheerful face greeted me.

'Hi,' I tried to hide the exhaustion. I tried to look pleased to see him.

'You're coming home soon, I hear,' he grinned.

'Oh yes!' I panicked. 'I'm coming home tomorrow.'

I hadn't bought any nappies.

'We won't have any nappies for the baby!' I exclaimed. 'John, you must go and buy some nappies and we'll need some sheets for the cradle, and blankets and ...'

'Er, I'll get a member of your choir to tell me what I need. After all, she's only a baby. She can't need that much. She's got her birthday suit already.' He picked up the bundle of baby rather clumsily. I was too exhausted to worry about his dropping her. He hadn't dropped her yet and there were nurses here, thank goodness. He looked down at the baby's little face.

'It can't be too difficult to get what she needs. The choir will be able to sort it.' There were dark rings under his eyes. He had not been sleeping much either. Penny wriggled and uttered one of her 'I'm winding up for a feed' squawks. He gave his bundle back to me quickly. 'I'll go home now and start ringing round.'

At 10 o'clock the next morning my case was packed. I was ready to go. The nurse who had helped me pack stood beside me.

'Here, you take the case,' I said to John as he walked towards me, the cool air from outside still emanating from his street clothes.

'No, I'll take the baby,' he grinned, stretching his arms forward.

'No, I can't carry anything heavy,' I said wearily. 'You take the case and *I'll* take the baby.' I put my arm well under the baby, holding her up to make sure she did not go near my operation scar, which was still very painful.

'Okay.' He lifted the case swiftly from the floor, knocking it on the side of the bed. I held the baby firmly.

'If you open the door with your other hand, I won't drop the baby,' I said as we reached the door. The nurse giggled behind us.

'Really, you two,' she said, walking closely behind us all the way outside.

As we drove into the village it took on a new look. The life-changing experiences I had had in hospital coloured my view of Sutton. The trees seemed greener, the streets dirtier. Could it be that I actually missed the antiseptic hospital environment?

As the car pulled into our drive I looked up.

'It's a baby girl!' was splashed all over our upstairs window.

'So the village knows about her now?' I smiled at John. He grinned back and opened the front door while I carried the baby inside. I gave her a quick feed, changed her and put her in the pram. Thank goodness we had something to change her into and something for her to lie down in. The choir had certainly been a help.

John fidgeted. 'I'll take her for a walk,' he said, grabbing hold of the pram and wheeling it outside. I looked briefly at his disappearing back, and crawled upstairs to bed for a lie down.

I woke with a start. The baby. Where was the baby? Wasn't it time for a feed? 'John?' I called. The house was silent. I struggled to my feet, walked carefully down the stairs and went outside into the sunshine.

'Have you seen John with the pram?' I yelled at the neighbour cleaning his car.

'No, sorry,' he replied giving the front offside light an extra polish.

I stormed up the street towards the village church with its pepper pot tower looming overhead. There was no sign of John and the pram. I called at every shop along the High Street. There was no sign of him. Sarah's. He might be at Sarah's. As I reached her front gate, there he was, standing in front of the pram in deep conversation, his hands gesticulating wildly.

'There you are! I've been looking all over the place for you!' I snapped. 'The baby needs feeding and changing. Didn't you realize?'

John looked blank. 'Anyway,' he continued to gesticulate to Sarah, 'it seems the wife has called. She who must be obeyed.' He took hold of the pram. I smiled weakly at Sarah. The baby squirmed uneasily. We hurried home.

I took on the role as 24-hour breast feeder, while John proudly told the village of his wonderful success. He was a father and proud to be one. I was exhausted. He was excited and had all sorts of plans for us to visit everyone and show them our new prize.

Chapter 16

The exhaustion never ceased. If I did not get some rest soon there would be an accident. I asked John to help and he agreed but nothing happened. Sometimes I asked him to change the baby and he would; at other times he had more important things that occupied his mind. I never understood what these important things were, but Penny remained unchanged. I dragged myself up and changed her. John remained in his world of indifference. Then, it came to a crisis. I *had* to get to sleep somehow.

John was sitting on the sofa. I clutched the baby, went over to him thrust the bundle onto his chest and said, 'Here, you take her. I'm going out in the car to get some sleep.' His eyes widened. He clutched the bundle nervously.

'But —' he started.

I didn't hear the rest. In a daze, I rushed out of the front door, slammed it behind me, and went to my car. My hands shook as I opened the door, put the keys into the ignition and started the engine. I forced my eyes open as I drove slowly out of the driveway. I turned left and drove to the nearest lay by, which was on the road to my previous work.

Peace, at last. I pulled the car up climbed onto the back seat, lay down and sleep, glorious sleep overcame me.

After about five minutes I was roused from my slumber by a loud tapping noise. Someone was tapping on the car window.

'What now!' I muttered. 'Can't I have my sleep?' The blurred face of a young man with a policeman's hat on looked at me. He indicated that I should wind the window down.

'Are you all right?' he looked straight into my bleary eyes.

'Yesh,' I murmured. 'I jusht wan sleep.'

'May I have your name and address?'

I couldn't believe it. Here I was, finally in a place where you'd think I would not be interrupted, and he wanted my name and address.

'Msss Wilks,' I slurred and stopped myself from snapping 'Now go away and let me get some sleep!'

'How do you spell your name?'

I could not believe it. What kind of cretin was he?

I forced myself to try to sound polite. 'W-i-l-k-s,' I said between gritted teeth.

He wrote it down slowly. My body swayed, ready to flop down into a sleeping position again. He stared into all the other seats of the car.

'The Wilks family,' he said knowingly. 'Any relation to Matthew Wilks?'

'I've no idea,' I stopped myself from adding 'and at the moment I could not care less'. In the back of my befuddled mind I thought the name sounded familiar. Where had I heard it before? I vaguely remembered something Taru had said when we stayed with her but a vision of John throwing the petrol can on the fire overtook my thoughts.

The policeman's voice became more insistent. 'What is your address, please?'

'My address?' What was it? For a moment I could not think. 'Oh, 2 Su'n Dri ...'

'All right,' he said writing it down, 'Now, why are you here?'

'I jush want some sleep,' I murmured. 'I've a new baby and I jush want to go to sleeeep.' I stopped myself from sliding down.

'Oh, a new baby, huh?' He grinned. I tried to force my lips to move into some kind of smile too. 'Well, if you are sure you're ...'

'Yesh, I'm fine I jush wan' some sleep.' I looked at him through my half-closed eyes. Finally he closed his notepad, tipped his hat, turned and left me alone.

'Sleep, sleep,' I murmured as I slumped down on the seat. After I had slept for a couple of hours, my eyes opened involuntarily. I stretched and yawned. Was the policeman real? Was I *really* questioned by the police or had I imagined it? And what did he mean that he knew our family already? Had John been committing a crime? No, I refused to believe it. His worst crime was loving his mother too much. Then what else? I sighed. Then I remembered. We had already met John's Uncle Matthew. It was Matthew Wilks who had made the name famous, or was it infamous? With a start, I realized I needed to get back to the baby. She must need another feed by now! Goodness knows what had happened while I slept. I would worry about Matthew Wilks and his girlfriend later.

It was a good six months before I saw light at the end of the tunnel. I was coping at last. The effects of the operation were not so severe. The baby would let me sleep for a few hours at least. But there was still no respite, no let-up. If I did not get out of the house I would go mad. The choir I had started gave me a glimpse of the world outside and I looked forward to a good sing on a Tuesday night. But this was not enough. If I didn't get the chance to have five minutes to myself, alone, without interruptions from baby or John, I would lose my mind.

'Would you mind if I went to work again?' I asked, when John and I were having an afternoon cup of tea.

'No,' John put his cup down. The baby was in her playpen between us. 'But I thought you wanted to be a stay-at-home mum?'

'So did I.' I poured some hot water into the teapot. 'That was until I found myself getting obsessed about the colour of the loo paper. I actually found myself changing it when it didn't match. Besides, I need a break, just five minutes to finish a cup of coffee on my own.'

On cue the baby cried. I put down the hot water jug and lifted her up. 'Time for a change then, eh?'

John stood up and put on his jacket. 'Well, I'll be off then. I'll go and see the Johnsons about next year's Feast.'

'You do that,' I called from upstairs, trying not to sound too annoyed. Why couldn't John change her? No, it was no good leaving things as they were. I needed a break and John was not the answer.

'I've got an interview with an agency next week,' I said as Babs and I stood in the sitting room. Penny was playing in her playpen between us and John was ensconced in his armchair with the newspaper.

Babs looked at Penny. 'Where do you think she got her red hair? Did anyone in your family have red hair?' She leaned over the playpen and handed Penny a rubber ring. Penny's little hand grabbed the ring and put it into her mouth. She would need feeding soon. I sat down on the sofa. There would be two more minutes at least before she would start to demand attention in earnest.

'No, not really. Uncle Sheridan had freckles, I remember that.'

Babs sat down next to me. 'What about John's family?' Babs and I looked at John who was sitting his armchair, the *Daily Telegraph* firmly hiding his features. He gave no response.

'John?' I asked, but there was still no response. I stood up slowly. Really, he could be so annoying! I stood over him and leaned over the newspaper until I could see his eyes. They were glued to the page. 'John,' I said loudly, 'did any of your relatives have red hair?'

John frowned.

'Red hair? Why is that important?' he asked, keeping his eyes firmly on the page.

'We want to know.'

John groaned and looked round the edge of the newspaper to spy Babs. He crackled the pages as he quickly pulled the paper towards his chest and leaned forward glaring at us.

'If you must know, I think there were a couple of aunts who had red hair but it's of no consequence, so let me get on with the paper. I've got to read the paper.' He shook the pages open and resumed reading.

I was tempted to ask why he thought he had to read the papers — it was not as if he were gainfully employed to read them — but thought better of it and returned to Babs.

'So it sounds as though it might be on John's side as he says a couple of aunts I've never heard of have red hair. I'd love to meet them,' I lowered my voice, 'but not now.' I mouthed to Babs, 'Not until John's in a better mood.' Babs nodded conspiratorially.

The following Friday, John bounded into the room. 'I made a good sale today,' he said as he came up behind me while I stood in the kitchen, clutching the cake tin I had just emptied. He gave me a quick hug, 'There'll be a good commission at Christmas.' He leaned over the cake I had just turned out, grabbed a knife from the drying up and cut himself a large slice. I ignored the crumbs that littered the floor — the floor was seriously in need of cleaning anyway.

'And we are going out to lunch on Sunday,' he said between mouthfuls.

My stomach turned. Not his mother's again. I could not stand it. I gripped the empty cake tin hard before letting it fall into the sink with a clatter.

'We have an invitation to go somewhere on Sunday?' I asked, praying that he did not recognize my fear that it would be to Mother-in-law's.

'Yes,' John said with his mouth full, 'to Luke and Irene Mason's house.'

My stomach calmed. I turned the taps on and water gradually filled the basin.

'Who are they?' I shouted loudly, to make myself heard above the water.

'Oh, they're customers I've known for years.' John used his loud public speaking voice. He could make himself heard above a herd of stampeding cattle if he wanted to. 'I often go there for lunch. Irene really wants to meet you.'

The cake tin was fully covered with water, so I turned the taps off, shook my hands and wiped them on my apron. I undid the apron strings and turned to face him. He had that boyish expression I remembered from the first day we met — full of mischief and determination, determined to wrench every vestige of fun out of the day.

'Would you like a cup of tea? Penny's sleeping upstairs.' I hung up the apron on the kitchen door. 'I see you've had your cake already.' We both grinned. Maybe now would be a good time to find out about his aunts.

'Yes, a cup of tea would be nice, and make it strong.' John dashed towards the stairs. 'I'll just phone Mother and tell her the good news.'

'You do that,' I muttered under my breath.

Half an hour later he came slowly down the stairs. His expression had lost some of its sparkle but there was still a glimmer of a smile on his lips.

'Your tea is ready. It's well and truly brewed, the way you like it. Shall I pour?'

'If you like.' John sat down.

I waited until he had had a good mouthful of tea and then, heart beating a little faster, I asked, 'Remember you mentioned your aunts may have red hair?' I tried to sound nonchalant, as though I was simply indulging in idle chat. I did not want him to clam up again. 'Do you mind if I ask who they are and where they live?'

John stared into his teacup. He fingered the handle. 'Oh, they're not important.' He paused to glance outside. Even he could not ignore the heavy silence that demanded an answer. 'I think they live somewhere near St Ives.' He leaned back in his chair holding his cup firmly, taking a sip and savouring the hot liquid.

'Are they your aunts on your mother's or your father's side?'

'My mother's,' he frowned, as if trying to forget an unpleasant truth.

'Have you met them?'

'Not really, I think I saw them from the distance when I was very little, at Granddad's funeral.'

'Well, did they have red hair?'

'I think so. What's it matter?'

'I find it interesting and one day I would like to be able to tell Penny where her red hair comes from.'

'Well, I'm not sure. I remember being more interested in the little sandwiches that had no crusts. Mother always made me eat the crusts at home. Any more tea?' He held out his cup expectantly.

I took his cup and saucer, poured in the milk and placed the tea strainer over it before lifting the cosy off the teapot and filling his cup again.

'Their surname would be the same as your mother's, right?'

'Yes.'

'What was your mother's maiden name again?' Mary and Bill had already mentioned the Cox family, but I could see it would no good pointing that out in this delicate conversation.

'Cox,' John scowled. 'Now, hand me the paper will you?'

'In a minute. Cox, you say. Was Audrey the name of the eldest sister?' I had no idea what their names were, but I was hoping to catch him unawares so that he revealed a name at least.

'Not Audrey,' he snapped, 'Gloria. Now hand me the newspaper, will you?' The tone was now harsh. I leaned forward quickly, took the newspaper off the arm of the sofa and handed it to him. He shook open the pages and sank back into the world of news and opinions of the day.

I sighed, finished my tea, left his on the table next to him and went to the kitchen to wash up. Well, I had found out one of their names at least. I could hardly wait until he had gone out to work or out to visit someone important, even his mother, so that I could get hold of one of the phone books that stood neatly in a line in his office upstairs. It would be easy to look up the name G. Cox in St. Ives.

Chapter 17

'I'll be out all day today,' John called as he made a dash for the car. He was anxious to leave before I could cross examine him about how long he intended to spend with his mother but for once I could hardly wait for him to go. Penny was fed, changed and asleep in her cot upstairs. Now for the phone book. I dashed into John's office, feeling guilty, as though even entering this room was breaking an unspoken rule. What was John's business was his and his alone but I shook off this fear and scanned the line of phone books. I was just about to pull the book from the shelf when I heard a key turn in the door. I gulped, dashed quickly into our room next to Penny's cot. My heart was beating fast. I waited for the heavy footsteps to sound on the stairs.

'I forgot something I promised to take Mother,' John called and I heard him rummage in the papers in the drawer downstairs. There was a pause but eventually the front door slammed as he went out again.

I counted to ten and then tentatively entered his office again. I paused. I could hear his car pull out of the drive. I pulled out the phone book and opened the pages. Appleton, Baker, Carrington ... ah here it is, 'Cox'. Penny gave a little winding-up whimper from her cot. Not now, Penny, not yet. 'G.Cox, 7 Heath St, St Ives.' It was there. It must be her. Should I phone? What would she make of a perfect stranger phoning? Would she want to hear from John and his family or was there something between them that should not be brought out in the open? My curiosity was too strong to ignore. I had to know. With one finger on the phone number I took the receiver off the hook and started to press the numbers. At that moment, Penny gave an unholy yell; she was well and truly awake and no matter how I tried to ignore her, now would not be the right time to phone. I hurriedly closed the book and returned it to the shelf, checked that I had not disturbed anything else in the room and went to Penny.

While I sat feeding Penny I tried to imagine what Gloria Cox looked like. Would she be like John or his mother? Maybe she would be a healthy version of John, full of fun, laughter and a zest for life. We could have a real family life, there would be no overwhelming feeling of isolation, Penny would have someone else who loved her and wanted to be a part of her upbringing. Oh, how I wished my mother had not died so young, and that my father was not on the other side of the world. How I wished for someone loving to be able to share my new role as mother.

Penny closed her mouth firmly. She had had enough food. I lifted her out of the high chair, checked to see if she needed changing and put her in her playpen. I looked at her little face. As I sat back and relaxed, watching Penny play with her toys, I thought of John's mother and her tirades of anger. Where did this anger come from? Would her sisters be the same? Would they create even more problems than we had already? I decided, no matter what, I would meet these sisters, with or without John. I had to know.

'Hurry *up!*' John called as he opened the front door.

'Getting Penny ready to go out is not something that you can do in a few seconds. What did you do with her coat?'

'What coat?'

'The one your had wrapped around her when you took her outside to see Mrs Miller over the road last night.'

'Oh, that one.'

'Well?'

John stood still for a moment, his hand resting on the door handle. 'In the kitchen, I think.'

Muttering under my breath, holding Penny firmly, I swept to the kitchen. On top of the kitchen table was her coat. I grabbed it and took Penny back to the front door.

'Nappies, food, change of clothes,' I muttered checking Penny's bag. The phone rang.

'Oh, for goodness sake, leave it! Let's go!' John snapped. I grabbed the bag, held Penny firmly and walked quickly to the car, ignoring the persistent ringing of the phone. John was seated in the front seat by now, the engine purring and his foot hovering over the accelerator. I flung open the passenger door to make sure John waited until everything was safely inside, and Penny was strapped in the back seat before we sped off to see the Masons.

'Have you got everything?' John asked as I slammed the passenger door shut and was putting the seat belt on.

'Yes,' I answered, hoping that Irene would be able to supply what I had probably forgotten.

The sun streamed into the car; my eyes smarted from the rays flashing through the trees as we sped out of the village. The trees were soon gone and the landscape stretched out on either side of the narrow road. I wondered who had been trying to reach us on the phone when we left so hurriedly. They could leave a message.

The land was chocolate brown, flat and bare. I clutched my seat. John focused on the narrow expanse ahead and, with experienced fingers, turned the wheel a fraction at a time to compensate for the bumps in the road as he negotiated the tiny lane. I glanced to our left and gripped the seat harder. One slip and we would soon be tumbling down into the marshy gap between the road and the land. I wondered how many deaths there had been on this road.

When we reached the junction, John checked for cars and swept confidently into the road turning right towards Earith.

'The washes are dry, notice,' said John, 'not like it was last winter.'

I murmured a positive reply, wondering what he was talking about. As we drove through the village of Earith some of the buildings looked familiar. The flatness of the land, the closeness of the houses and the occasional mansard roof reminded me of the few houses I had seen in Holland on my travels when I was single. It seemed so long ago. I leaned over towards the back seat to check on Penny. She sat comfortably asleep.

The sign to Needingworth was again familiar.

'We've been this way before, haven't we?' I said.

'Yes, you remember, I took you to the Old Ferry Boat Inn?'

'Oh yes, how could I forget? That was wonderful.' And Mother-in-law was there too, I thought. It was so long ago. I closed my eyes and tried to picture the huge oak beams that stretched above the dining room, the whole place reeking of history, a history that was far earlier than anything I had ever come across in Tasmania and a history that already seemed to have distanced itself from my life in the more troubled present.

'Where do the Masons live?'

'In Hemingford Grey,' John replied.

My heart skipped a beat. One of the road signs said 'St Ives'. I clenched my fingers. This must be where the Cox sisters lived.

'Was that a sign for St Ives?' I ventured, trying not to sound too interested.

'I suppose so,' John frowned, as if concentrating hard on the next junction.

'When I was going to St Ives, I met a man with seven wives ...' I started the well-known nursery rhyme.

'That's St Ives in Cornwall, nothing to do with here,' John said abruptly.

'Nevertheless, have we been to this St Ives before?' I asked. I knew we hadn't but today was the day I was determined to solve something of the mystery aunts. If I played my cards right, we would at least find out where they lived today and maybe even call on them...

'No,' John snapped, an edge of finality in his tone.

'Will we get a chance to look at it today?' I tried to keep the tone light and casual.

'I doubt it. We're late for lunch with the Masons as it is.' He closed his mouth tightly, his face assuming that 'don't dare push me any further' look. I didn't.

'Isn't it pretty!' I exclaimed as we entered the village of Hemingford Grey. I had never before seen so many thatched cottages, side by side. The white stucco of the walls, the narrow streets and the air of a sleepy village untouched by the changing times made me wish I had brought a camera. I glanced at John, but even if I had brought one to take a lasting picture of this charming village, now would not have been the time to try to persuade John to stop; we were late already. Besides, I knew that if we stopped even for a second, little Penny's head would have lifted immediately and sustenance and a nappy change would be required. I sighed and watched the road turn towards the next junction. John turned hard left and we entered a nondescript estate, rows of look-alike brick buildings of a much more modern era. We pulled up directly outside number 11, the number painted on the garage door. The front door swept open and a small woman with a shock of golden curls smiled broadly at us. She rushed to John as he climbed out of his seat and gave him a huge hug.

'Welcome, welcome,' she gushed, 'we're so pleased you came. Are you going to introduce us to your fine lady?'

John grinned and, with his voice breaking with emotion, said, 'This is my wife, Sally. Sally, meet Irene and Luke.' Luke, by now, had crept up behind his wife, grinning broadly. He smiled and shook my hand without uttering a single word. Irene had said all that needed to be said.

'Ooh, and this must be Penny,' Irene crooned as she leaned over the seat and peered into the back of the car. Penny's head had shot up the moment the car stopped and she was making a good effort to drown out everyone with her cries. Irene looked at the scrunched-up face and wide screaming mouth.

'Isn't she gorgeous?' she lied. 'Bring her inside. You must want to see to her, Sally. I've prepared a room for you upstairs.'

John suddenly opened the back door to the car and lifted Penny out. I heaved a sigh of relief. Visiting was a good idea — John seemed particularly attentive to our needs when there were friends to impress. I pursed my lips, chastising myself for such an unkind thought.

'Thank you, John' I said, and smiled weakly at Irene. 'Would you mind if I went straight upstairs first then?'

'Of course you must, and we'll have time to talk farming and to remind John of his misspent youth while you're there.' John gave me Penny and Irene led me into her sparkling house. As we rushed upstairs I briefly glimpsed rows of shiny brasses, a highly polished table and chairs and shepherd boy and girl ornaments filling a wide mantelpiece.

'In here, Sally,' Irene said as stepped aside and waved me into a large spare room with double bed and embroidered chair. 'You can change Penny there and I have some rusks downstairs for her to chew. We'll leave you to it, Sally. Is there anything you want before I go downstairs?'

I shook my head.

'The bathroom is the first door on your right,' Irene called as she went downstairs.

I dealt with Penny's dirty nappy, and was eventually seated on the embroidered chair with Penny on my knee. I leant back savouring the few moments of peace, and time alone with our first-born. She really was a marvel. Her red hair looked darker than usual in the dimmed light of the room. I thought of the mystery sisters. Irene seemed friendly enough; perhaps she knew them? I decided to make no definite plans, but if the opportunity came...

'John, help Sally bring Penny downstairs, there's a dear,' Irene said to him amicably as she watched me step carefully down the stairs, clutching Penny closely. 'Bring her here and put her on this mat. There's plenty of room.' She pointed to a small mat placed in the corner to the side of their large sitting room. There was a pile of toys in the centre of it. The dining room table shone in the sunlight, the table set for many courses for four people, with a highchair placed at the end.

'You come and sit by me, John,' Irene patted the seat next to her as John finished putting Penny down. I went and hovered by Penny. She started crawling towards the bookshelves. I leant down and picked her up immediately.

'Don't worry, Sally, bring her to the table and we can take it in turns to hold her. In fact, can I hold her now?' I could see Irene could hardly wait. I handed over the squirming bundle and Penny calmed immediately as Irene put her on her lap and tickled Penny's tummy with hands that had had years of experience. 'Luke will dish, won't you dear?'

Luke, his stolid frame unmoved, nodded with the earnestness of a seasoned caterer. He stood at the head of the table, sharpened the carving knife with considerable gusto and was soon slicing the red beef, deftly passing out the laden plates. He dished out the piping hot vegetables that he collected from the kitchen until we were all satisfied.

'I think she is hungry,' Irene said as Penny reached for her plate. 'I'll put her in the high chair, if that's all right? She can share my dinner.' She looked at me to see if I agreed. I nodded vigorously. It was a pity Irene was not related.

Luke sat down, raised a glass of red wine, we all chorused 'Cheers' and the phone rang.

Chapter 18

The phone continued to ring. No one seemed to take any notice. Luke began to stand

'Leave it, Luke,' Irene said firmly. 'If it is important, they will leave a message and nothing can be so serious that it cannot wait until we have finished our meal'. Luke smiled and sat down again.

'You're right, dear. They can wait.' His voice was deep and the vowels were wide — as though filled with sunshine and the fresh air of the countryside. I warmed to him immediately. I wondered about the phone call we had ignored. Had we told anyone that we were coming here?

'How is your mother, John?' Irene turned to John. I forced a smile as John began to list the woes his mother had been suffering this week. She had felt so excluded from our lives that she had felt obliged to go away on a short holiday. 'I persuaded her to let me pay for it,' he concluded.

I sat up straight. He had never discussed this with me. We could not afford our own holiday. How could we afford to pay for a holiday for his mother, of all people? Did John not realize this? At least I knew now that John would be picking her up next Friday when she returned. I continued to force my smile while I made a mental note not to cross examine him next Friday about where he had been and to have a good look at our joint bank account to work out how we were going to pay off some of our debts.

'You have had a hard time of it, haven't you?' Irene patted John's hand. 'You know you should keep in contact with the rest of her family — even if she doesn't want you to. Someone needs to keep an eye on the older folk. She would soon forgive you, you know, and then she might not feel so lonely.'

John paled, his lips tightened and he focused on his meal.

Irene bit her lip, paused and turned her attention to me.

'I believe you are from Tasmania?'

'Yes,' I managed to say after a pause while I finished chewing and swallowed a rather nicely done baked potato.

'You must miss it very much. Is it very different from here?'

'Yes, it is, but I love it here — there is so much history and such a strong sense of tradition, something we seriously lack in Tasmania.'

'Well if you are interested in history, you must go to St Ives. Have you taken her to St Ives yet?' she asked John.

John frowned. 'No, not yet. We don't really have time now that we have a baby.'

'Nonsense,' Irene said, the word no more that a gentle admonishment. 'After lunch, and after Sally and Penny have had a little rest, we can all go and explore St Ives. We have a package to drop off there anyway. You would like that, wouldn't you, Sally?'

'Oh, yes please, I would love it.' I could hardly believe my luck. John looked down at his empty plate.

156

'We'll lead and you two follow in your car,' Irene called as she stood next to their Rover. 'After we've dropped off the package, we'll park near the little bridge so that we can go for a walk by the river and then come back for a cup of tea.' Irene shouted above the noise of the Rover engine as Luke eased the car out of their garage.

John strapped Penny into the back seat and opened the car door for me. I sat very still, not daring to speak. Tight-lipped, John climbed into the car, put his seatbelt on and started the engine. 'I don't know why we're going to St Ives,' he said unhappily. 'There's not really much to see — just the tiny one-way bridge and a statue of that traitor, Oliver Cromwell.' I said nothing.

The Masons' green Rover moved steadily ahead, past the signpost for St Ives, and took a turning to the right. We were in St Ives.

'Where *are* they going?' John said, anxiety obvious in his rising tone.

'I think they said they have to deliver a package,' I reminded him. 'They said they would do that first, remember?'

'But not here, why *here*?' John's tone was dark and anxious, too anxious. I was puzzled. Why should he be so anxious? Then I saw the name of the road we were about to turn into: 'Heath Road'. My heart thumped. This was the very same road that his aunts lived in. What number was it again? Seven, I was sure it was seven. Did the Masons know the aunts? Maybe they were delivering a package to them? After all, they knew John's mother and surely she must contact her sisters sometimes, even if she refused to speak about them. Maybe the package was from her? I tried to calm my racing pulse. It was all very unlikely. It was too much of a coincidence. One, three, five ...I clutched the seat under me. The Masons' car pulled up outside Seven. It was the aunts' place!

Luke walked up the straight stone path and banged the brass knocker on the door three times. The house was one of the older houses in the estate, large faded yellow brick and semi-detached. The path ran beside a closely cropped lawn; a round bush stood next to the door. Everything in its place just like Eunice's, I thought.

Luke looked back towards Irene who was tapping on John's window.

'Come on,' she shouted through the window, 'all of you. Come on and meet the Coxes. We'll only be here for a minute.'

John reluctantly left his seat, glumly came round to my side, opened my door and extricated Penny from the back seat. Penny's red head lifted up and she looked at her daddy, only curious, not fractious for a change.

A cool breeze had sprung up, ruffling our hair. Luke's thin wisp lifted up in the wind to reveal his perfectly round bald head. He looked vulnerable, innocent, adorable, I thought. The door opened a crack.

'Yes?' a thin, penetrating voice asked.

'Miss Cox, it's Irene and Luke delivering your birthday present. It was your birthday last week, wasn't it?'

'Why, yes, I suppose it was,' the thin voice replied. The door opened a little more. Irene stepped forward. I almost expected her to put her foot firmly through the opening in the doorway in case it was shut again, but she didn't.

'I've brought some people to meet you, too' she called through the gap.

'You have?' The voice sounded a little perturbed.

'*Do* let us in,' Irene begged. 'It's cold out here and Luke is dying for a cup of tea.' Luke looked at me, eyebrows lifted arms out, the picture of innocence.

'Oh, yes, Luke.' The door opened fully. 'I suppose you had better come in. Take your shoes off.' I saw a full head of curly red hair retreat into the house as Irene, Luke and the rest of us followed.

The hallway was dark, the wallpaper faded as though it had not been changed or painted since the house was first built. I wished I had insisted that John wore a new pair of socks — his toe was clearly visible on his right foot.

We filed into a large room at the end of the corridor. A tall grandfather clock ticked loudly from the corner of the room. A huge sofa and several large armchairs filled the remaining space. An old-fashioned fireplace was hidden by a large screen that had some red roses embroidered on its face. I wondered if the sisters had made it. One of the armchairs stirred. A small frail woman leaned out of the chair to look at us, her features pinched with starvation rather than ill humour, her thin red hair cropped short, her long thin fingers stretching out to shake our hands.

'This is Hannah,' the first red-haired lady spoke, her voice exactly the kind of voice you would expect from someone so tall and slender who was putting on a brave face, feigning command of herself and her environment. I guessed she must be Gloria. She had Eunice's eyes, and apparent dominance, but the cold hurt feelings that Eunice emanated were not there. This face was warm and welcoming in an assured but humble way.

'Sit down,' she said and took her place in the armchair opposite her sister, both chairs either side of the fireplace. Irene and Luke sat on the sofa and Irene waved her hand at John and me, beckoning us to sit. I sat down on the thin upright chair next to Irene and hoped it would hold my heavy weight. John plonked Penny down on the floor in front of the only remaining armchair, put her nappy bag behind the door and sat down, bolt upright.

'You remember John, Eunice's son, don't you Gloria?' Irene asked.

Gloria leaned forward to look more closely at him. Her smooth face broke out into a smile. 'Why yes, yes, you must be John. It's a very long time since I last saw you.' She put her hand forward as if to stroke him. 'My, haven't you grown into a handsome young man. Just like your father.' She withdrew her hand and paused for a moment. Then, as if she suddenly remembered something, she sparked up and looked at me, 'This must be your wife', and looked at Penny, who was playing with the hem of the armchair cover, 'and your first child.' She smiled warmly towards us.

John cleared his throat. 'This is Sally and Penny.' He waved his hand in our direction as though we were inadvertent interlopers.

I smiled, glancing at John to see how enthusiastically I should react. His face was still and unreadable. I kept my gentle smile. Penny wriggled towards her dad.

'Irene has told me so much about you all,' Gloria said. 'I am *so* glad you have come. Hannah, tea for everyone.'

'Do bring the little one closer to me,' Gloria asked John, who stood up and obliged. 'What lovely hair she has. Just the same as yours, Hannah, do you think?'

By now Hannah was on her feet and cooing over Penny as well.

'Perhaps, although I think she has the same auburn tint as you, and the same curls.'

'She is lovely,' Gloria said to John and me, 'may I hold her?'

John stood up. 'I don't ...'

'Of course you can,' I interrupted, lifting up Penny and putting her firmly onto Gloria's lap. Penny fingered the buttons on Gloria's blouse. Gloria glowed. 'Oh she really *is* lovely. If only — '

Hannah was on her feet. 'Now don't start, Gloria. It's all in the past — water under the bridge — over and done with. We don't want to be talking about it now, not to John and Sally. Can I hold the baby?' she asked, looking at me. I nodded, wondering what she meant by 'it's all in the past'. What was all in the past? I opened my mouth to ask but felt John's eyes glaring at me. I closed my mouth.

By now Hannah was cuddling Penny closely, swaying gently, with Penny comfortable in her arms. Penny snuggled in appreciatively. I grinned proudly. For once Penny was doing the right thing. Suddenly Penny leaned back screwed up her face, and regurgitated a little of her undigested food from dinner over Hanna's hand and onto the pale carpet. I grabbed a couple of nappies from the bag behind the door. 'I am *so* sorry,' I blurted, handing one to Hannah and taking Penny from her quickly. I mopped down Penny's front and brushed the carpet. Thank goodness she had not eaten much at dinner.

'Oh, it's all right. Although I have never had children of my own, I am an expert babysitter and in that sense have had hundreds of babies to hold before.' She reassured me and sat down, as if nothing untoward had happened. 'Are you all right now, little one?' She handed me the nappy and stroked Penny under the chin. Penny gurgled happily. I stuffed the dirty nappies into the bag behind the door.

'So, how are you both?' Irene asked. 'Have you got your coal supplies in for the winter? Do you have any little jobs you would like Luke to do?'

'No, no, we're all right,' said Gloria, 'You have done so much for us already.' She paused nervously. 'Er, have you seen Eunice lately?' She looked at her fingers that were now clutched on her knees.

'Yes, she's all right. You have no need to worry,' Irene soothed.

'But we do worry,' said Hannah. 'Ever since...'

'Not in front of John and Sally, remember?' Gloria interrupted, glaring hard at her sister.

'What not in front of John and me?' I blurted more loudly than intended, making Penny stare at me with this unexpected outburst. I had had enough of secrets. It was time the truth was out. If it was all in the past, what harm could it do to us now? I did not dare look at John. 'I would be very grateful if you could tell us a little more about John's past.' I forced my tone to sound calmer, more approachable 'He seems so confused about it and I want to be able to tell Penny all about the family she has missed.' Holding Penny firmly, I lowered my head, pleading with each of the sisters in turn.

'Well,' Hannah said as she stood up, holding Penny firmly. 'It happened so long ago, even before John was born.'

'I do not agree with this!' Gloria snapped. 'I'll get the tea as you seem to have forgotten!' She stood up, her height increased even further with her indignation. She stepped solidly and firmly out of the room and down the corridor to where I presumed the kitchen must be.

'I'll help you.' Irene stood up. 'Come on, Luke, you come too.' With that, Irene and Luke left the room. We could hear Gloria's heavy shoes striking the paving stones, above the lighter steps of Irene and Luke as they processed away from the sitting room. John sat in his armchair pale, sullen and quiet. I put Penny on the floor and leaned forward assuming my pleading position. Hannah blushed.

'I'm not sure,' Hannah's hands tightened. Penny pulled at the armchair cover.

'That's enough!' John leapt to his feet. 'We do not want to hear any more about it.' He snatched Penny up from the floor. Penny squawked.

'Here,' he said and thrust Penny at me. I held her firmly, cuddling her and swinging her gently to and fro until she calmed. Hannah shrugged, holding her hands out to me. What could she do? The grandfather clock ticked loudly in the tense silence that remained until we could hear the rattle of teacups advancing down the hallway.

163

Chapter 19

I sat glumly in the car, thinking how to broach the subject I really wanted to discuss.

'The Masons were lovely. I hope we can see them again' I said as lightly as I could 'but why didn't you let Hannah tell us about your mother?'

'It's none of your business,' John snapped. 'Anyway, you've seen the aunts now, so I hope you're satisfied.' He put his foot down further on the accelerator. The car bounced suddenly on the Fenland road.

I bit my lip. It would have to wait for another time. I would wait until he was out again and maybe arrange another meeting with the aunts — perhaps with Hannah, as she was the one who just might tell me what had gone on before. I would find out what had happened whether he wanted me to or not. Perhaps it would explain something about this other John that was emerging as he reacted so badly and so strongly to things that should not matter to him at all. What did it matter so much what happened in the past? Even though I was determined to find out more about what happened in the past, whatever I discovered would not shake our relationship. I married him, not his mother, his aunts or his past. Surely he understood this? The pepper-pot church of Sutton came into view. I sighed. Another baby-ruled night was ahead.

As we pulled up in our drive, Penny started complaining. She was tired and hungry, like me, I thought. I climbed out of the car, opened Penny's door, extricated her from her car seat and went to the front door. I rummaged in my pocket, withdrew the keys and opened the door. Penny cried. I rushed her inside and as I dashed her upstairs to change her I could see the light flashing on our answer phone.

I brought Penny downstairs, took her into the kitchen, gave her a rusk and turned to see John grinning.

'It was your father,' he smiled. 'He's fine. In fact he's coming over next month to see us all.' I grinned. Dad, coming here? At last I would have someone I could confide in, someone who understood me and would understand.

The following Tuesday, I had my chance to see if I could meet up with Hannah and find out what had happened between the sisters so long ago. I was sure it had something to do with what was troubling John.

'I have a conference in London tomorrow,' John had informed me over dinner the night before. 'I'll be back very late, so don't get me any dinner. I'll get it in London before I return'. He put his knife and fork together on his plate. 'We are meeting at a hotel near Harrods, so I may pop in and see what I can get Penny, OK?'

'Fine,' I said absently. He gave me a look of surprise and stood up. At that moment, I could not have cared what he was going to spend on the new baby. Our debts were so high anyway. I was caught up in the thought that the next day would be the day to arrange a meeting with Hannah. I could hardly wait.

Monday night took forever to pass. Penny woke up only once but after I had seen to her I saw every hour on the clock until 6 a.m. when John's alarm went off. I was feeding Penny when he got out of bed, got dressed, grabbed some cereal for breakfast, gave me a hasty peck on the cheek and dashed out of the front door.

The house was quiet. It was only 6.30 in the morning. It was too early. I had changed Penny and put her down to sleep again and it was still too early — 7.15 a.m. I got dressed slowly, made my own breakfast and took my tea into the sitting room. I heard the milkman's van clatter along the road in front of our house. He was late today. The milk bottles rattled on the doorstep. I would let the poor man escape before I grabbed the milk bottles he had just delivered. I watched the neighbours leave for work one after the other.

Penny called from upstairs. I brought her down and put her in her playpen. At 8 a.m. I collected the milk bottles but it was still a little early. I watched Penny's red curls bob up and down as she crawled around her playpen and I thought about John's redheaded aunts. The sisters looked as though they were fully retired by now, so they probably wouldn't start functioning until 9 o'clock. At 8.45 I could stand it no longer. I ran to the office, grabbed the phone book and dialled the Cox number. My heart was racing. Please let it be Hannah who answers, please.

'Hello?' the voice was tentative.

'Hello' I said, clearing my throat before I spoke again, 'It's Sally Wilks here. Do you remember we called on Sunday?'

'Oh yes, of course. How are you? How is little Penny?'

'We're fine,' I said hurriedly, still not sure if I was talking to Hannah or Gloria. 'Is that Hannah I am speaking to?'

'Why yes, dear, of course. Gloria is out in the garden at the moment, putting out some more seed for the birds. Can I help you?'

'Yes, yes,' I took in a deep breath. 'I wondered if you would like to come to Ely and perhaps meet up for coffee sometime?'

'I would love to. Gloria would love to as well. Would you like both of us to come?

'Well, yes, although maybe it would be best if you came alone. I feel so shy and I find when there are more than two ladies having coffee together it can be difficult sometimes to get a word in edgeways.' I grimaced. How lame could an excuse be!

'I see,' said Hannah, who understood everything I had intended. 'I have to go. I can hear Gloria outside the back door. I'll meet you at the Lamb Hotel at 11 o'clock on Thursday. I'll tell her I have to go to Ely Library for a special book and that I want to get some things from the market. All right?'

'Yes, yes thank you!' The phone clicked. Hannah had gone. I put the receiver down, clutched my arms round my body and danced around the room. I accidentally bumped into some of John's papers on the desk and they fell in a huge heap on the floor. I had done it now. I stopped, open-mouthed. He would know I had been in his office! I frantically gathered up the papers and tried to put them back the way I had seen them earlier, but I could not remember if they were in the same order. I bit my lip. I would have to admit that I had been in his office.

Penny squawked. I dashed downstairs. Penny's squawk was a cry of pleasure as she had found something new to do with the flexible clown.

I thought of Hannah telling a white lie to Gloria. But maybe she would not be telling a lie, maybe she *did* need a book from Ely Library and that she wanted some things from the market. It sounded as if she may have been there before. Maybe I too had to go to the library, to find out more about evening classes, and then the market in Ely. When I had wanted to go to work I had mentioned that I might do some evening classes too. Maybe it was time for me to take up something new. It would be quite natural for me to go to the library to ask for information. I breathed out. It was all right. Everything would be fine. I picked up Penny and hugged her until she squirmed and wanted to get back to her toys. I put her down and faced the huge pile of clothes that needed washing.

Thursday morning finally arrived and Penny was particularly slow in feeding. How did she do it? No matter how hard I tried to get her to fit into any plans of mine, she managed to thwart them, time and time again. You could almost be sure. If it wasn't Penny, it would be John, but today John was all right. He was going to his mother's to take her shopping. She had wrenched her arm or something. I nearly forgot to sound disgruntled when he said he was going to see his mother. At least I remembered not to sound too enthusiastic when I said, 'I suppose if she has damaged her arm, she will need you to help her quite a bit.' I grimaced as I remembered how John had glanced up at me at that moment, unsure if I was being sarcastic or not.

'No, no', I protested, 'I really mean it. It's not as if she's making it up or anything. Honestly, John, I wish her no harm and if she has hurt herself — 'I gulped. I wished I had not said 'if'. 'I mean to say, now that she *has* hurt herself, of course you must go and help her — even overnight if you need to.' I took a breath, glancing in his direction. Was he buying it? I decided to add, 'But *do* try to come home as soon as you can.' I crossed my fingers behind my back, hoping the last sentence was spoken with the ring of truth that I had intended.

'Well, thank you,' John grinned, hardly believing his luck. 'I probably won't need to stay overnight, but I might stay and have tea with her.'

'All right then,' I said as begrudgingly as I could.

The sky was grey. It had rained early in the morning but the clouds were no longer heavy with water. It would probably not rain again, but I decided to take Penny's waterproof cover and my umbrella to be on the safe side. Thank goodness I had persuaded John that I, too, needed a car so that I could get Penny to the hospital if he was away at a conference (or at his mother's, I had quietly muttered to myself).

I strapped Penny in the back, climbed into the driver's seat and turned on the engine. I smiled. It was a beauty. It always started first time. I revved the engine a little to let the choke do its job. I was just in time. It would take me 10 minutes to drive to Ely and as long as I found a place to park fairly quickly, I would be at the Lamb Hotel to meet Hannah Cox at 11 o'clock. I was about to check behind me before driving off when I heard a loud tapping on my window. What now?

Mrs Miller, her eagle eyes darting from me to the baby, waved her hand up and down. She was not going to move until I wound the window down. I forced a smile.

'Mrs Miller, what can I do for you?'

'My, hasn't Penny grown,' she cooed. I kept my hands on the wheel and revved the engine a little again. 'Oh,' she said, realizing that I was not going to stop, 'a parcel has been delivered to me by mistake. Just wait there a minute and I'll bring it to you.'

'But —'

Mrs Miller didn't hear me. I watched her back retreating slowly as she shuffled across the road to her house, her slippers getting damper by the minute on the wet road surface. I prayed that I would not develop a humped back like that when I got older, or maybe she had been born with it? I drummed my fingers on the steering wheel. She eventually emerged from her faded yellow door and, clutching the parcel, she shuffled towards the car.

'It's addressed to John, but I am sure I can give it to you to give to him, all right?' She held the parcel just out of my reach. She hesitated.

'Yes, it's perfectly all right,' I snapped, leaning as far as I could out of the window, snatching the parcel, and flinging it onto the seat next to me. 'Thank you, *so* much. I'm sorry, must go. I'll probably see you when I get back,' I shouted as I revved the car very loudly.

Mrs Miller finally took the hint, stepped back onto the damp grass and watched me drive hurriedly into the street and round the corner. I did not dare look back. I refused to feel guilty about rebuffing the kind lady. I would make it up to her tomorrow — invite myself round for coffee, taking Penny, too of course.

There was a parking space opposite Woolworth's. I quickly grabbed the pushchair from the boot and opened it out. I unstrapped Penny, who looked very much awake and curious, and placed her into the pushchair, then put my umbrella and Penny's waterproof cover in the bottom of the chair and wheeled her up the hill towards town. The hill seemed steeper than I remembered. The street was crowded. I stopped for a second to look at my watch. I was just in time if I hurried. I clambered into the hotel, the pushchair making a racket as I struggled to get it over the doorstep, and went into the bar area. I spotted Hannah's short red hair in an armchair at the back of the room. I smiled and wheeled Penny towards her.

'I'm so glad you came,' I said as I pecked her on the cheek. We were related, weren't we? I parked Penny next to me. Penny was still wide-awake but not hungry yet, thank goodness. She sat contented, banging her little fists against the toys I had strung to the front of her chair.

'I'll get the coffees, shall I?' Hannah pushed her handbag into the corner of her chair, unclipped it, took out her purse and turned towards the bar. I made a protesting noise but it was apparent to both of us that it made sense if she got the coffees. 'Milk and sugar?' she asked.

'Yes, please.' I would have agreed to milk and arsenic if she had asked. I was in a hurry to find out the family secret that had caused so much trouble.

I looked out of the hotel window while Hannah stood at the bar waiting to be served. There were a lot of farmers and their wives going to market today. Then I saw them. My mouth dropped open. I could recognize those heads anywhere. Oh no! There, walking in front of the window was John with Eunice firmly attached to his arm. Her other arm was in a sling. John was gesticulating wildly towards her. Her lips were firmly closed and she was looking down. I ducked my head down. Please, no! I prayed that they were not coming into the hotel! My hurried pulse thundered in my ears. I took in a deep breath and focused. I lifted my head slightly. They were moving slowly forwards, too engrossed in their argument to look in the window. Silly, I chastised myself as I sat up; they were not even heading in the right direction. They were not coming into the hotel. They were going towards the market. I decided I would have to phone the library for the information about courses I could do, lie about there being anything I wanted at the market and make a hasty retreat home. But then, why was I so afraid? It would not matter if they saw Penny and me — we were perfectly entitled to go to the market. But what if they saw Hannah? As long as they did not see us together, it would be all right. If they saw Hannah alone, they would ignore her as usual. I stood up and sat in the seat with my back to the window just to be on the safe side.

Hannah arrived back at the table, both hands holding cups of steaming coffee, her purse wedged firmly under her arm. I leaned forward, grabbed her handbag from her chair and shoved it into the seat next to me.

'You might want to sit here, with your back to the window,' I said hurriedly before she sat down, 'I have just seen Eunice and John.'

'Oh no!' she said, rattling the cups so the contents spilled into the saucers.

'No, it's all right. They were walking away from the hotel towards the market. It would take them ages to get back here, even if they decided to call in. Besides, as long as they don't see us together, it will be OK.'

'Oh dear,' said Hannah, her cheeks pale, her hands trembling. I rescued one of the cups before it lost all of its contents.

'Is this mine?' I asked, trying to take her mind off my sighting.

'Oh yes,' she said, 'I'm sorry, I've spilled it, I'll go and get —'

'It's fine, it's fine,' I said quickly. 'We'd better have a quick conversation and go, just in case they do want to come in. Please, please tell me what the problem is between you and Gloria and Eunice.'

Chapter 20

Hannah sat precariously on the edge of her seat, her hand still clutching her cup and saucer, her thumb drenched by the coffee that had spilled into the saucer.

'It's difficult,' she said, biting her lip. I pursed my lips, forcing myself to wait. Some more people walked into the room. We turned our heads sharply. It was an old man, his ruddy face and rapid stride evidence of his hours outside on his farm. His plump wife, clutching a basket full of goodies, followed behind.

'Well?' I asked looking straight into Hannah's hazel eyes.

She gulped. 'It all happened so long ago.' She sipped her coffee, grimacing. By now the coffee had turned cold. 'Before John was born.'

'Yes?' I strongly resisted the urge to shake her. I knew this already.

'His dad was such a lovely man.' She smiled, whirling the contents of her coffee around as she thought back to their earlier days.

'Yes?' Penny's little feet drummed her chair. I pushed it backwards and forwards quickly. Not now, Penny, not now. I stopped and handed her the menu to play with, not caring what she did with it. The information Hannah was about to give me was too important.

'Well —' Hannah leaned forward, lowering her voice to just above a whisper, 'John's dad was once engaged to Gloria, you know.'

'Really? What happened?' I ignored the sound of tearing paper that came from Penny's pushchair.

'I would hate to say anything against Eunice, but I'm sure she was the mystery girlfriend who had already persuaded John's father's brother, Matthew, to steal from his company.'

'Eunice, the mystery girlfriend?' My, she did put it about! I sat back in my chair. I tried to picture John's mother as a mistress and had to admit she was slim and graceful. She did seem to know how to get her own way.

'Unfortunately,' Hannah grimaced, 'all the evidence was against him. I would not put it past her —' She looked at me sadly. She knew she did not need to finish her sentence. I understood immediately how the gracious Eunice could well have planted the evidence.

'That's awful!' I said. 'It must have been terrible for you, being her sisters, to think that she could do such a thing.'

'It got worse.' Hannah sipped her coffee. 'Getting Matthew jailed was not enough. After that – ' she paused. Then as if she had suddenly made up her mind, she blurted, 'Then she upset Gloria too.'

'Yes?' an impatient tone edged my voice.

'Well, there is no other way to say it,' Hannah pouted. 'Once Matthew was jailed, Eunice stole Walter from Gloria when she had to go away to look after Aunty Flo and that's all there is to it!' She put her coffee cup down on the table and sat back in her chair, her eyes glistening, her hands clutching her coat front indignantly.

'But —' I searched her face and decided to risk it. 'But if he was truly in love with Gloria, he didn't have to give in to Eunice.'

'There was more to it.'

I raised an eyebrow.

'Eunice, in a fit of spite, said she was going to do her utmost to capture Walter's heart while Gloria was away and she succeeded. She got pregnant. Walter swore that the baby was not his child but he did the right thing by her. When she said she was pregnant, he did not really believe her, but because he *had* been unfaithful to Gloria once, only once — when he had had a bit too much to drink in the New Year — he had no other choice. They got married. It was a sad, sad day.'

'So John is actually illegitimate?' I asked incredulously.

'No, no, she lost that baby — well she *says* she lost the baby, and your John was the first child they had after they were married.'

'But then surely it's Gloria who should not be speaking to Eunice, not the other way round?'

'That's the problem. It has always been the problem. Eunice has always been jealous of us. No matter what we do to try to make her feel better, she will have none of it.'

'Maybe it's because she feels guilty?'

'Maybe, but every time we try to heal the breach she refuses to speak to us. She is a very troubled woman who is using John as her prop.'

'Maybe if I talk to John and he talks to her?'

'Oh, people have been talking to her. She has even been in the care of a psychiatrist.' Hannah suddenly clutched my hand. 'Please don't tell John I told you this. Nobody but Eunice, Gloria and I know of this. It's just like it was with Jim, only worse.' She suddenly put her hand up to her mouth.

'Jim?'

'No,' Hannah said sharply, 'no, that's enough.' She grabbed her handbag and stood up. 'Now I must go so that I can go to the market and the library. I have said enough. Oh, I do hope I don't see Eunice and John.'

Hannah moved swiftly towards the doorway. 'Give me a ring sometime. I'd love to keep in contact, although only ring on Wednesdays when Gloria is out, eh?' She dashed through the doorway and outside. I sat dumbfounded and watched her little figure scurry towards the market, her head down and her shoulders hunched.

'Poor Hannah, poor Gloria, poor Matthew,' I sighed, as I looked at the shreds of paper littering the floor beneath Penny's chair. Penny spluttered, waving her hands about, frustrated with the damp pieces of the menu that persisted in sticking to her mouth. I started to extricate the pieces of paper. Jim? I wonder who Jim was and why did she say it was just like it was with Jim, only worse?

I hurriedly gathered up the other pieces of paper, gave Penny's mouth a quick wipe with my fingers, stuffed the remains of the menu into my pocket, turned the pushchair round and pushed it out of the door without a single glance at the staff. I hoped they would not recognize me again. I just had time to make an appointment at the bank and grab some vegetables. I prayed I would not bump into John and his mother, not today.

When I arrived home, John was standing outside talking to Mrs Miller.

'Ah, here she is.' Mrs Miller walked quickly to the car and leaned over to look at the back seat.

'Have you been on an outing, little one?' she asked Penny, who stared at her blankly.

John opened my door. 'I believe you have a package for me?'

'Yes,' I said hurriedly, 'It's still here on the seat next to me.' I pulled it out from under my coat and gave it to him. He took it and started to open it.

'Can you get Penny out for me?' I asked.

'Oh, yes,' he said absently, put the parcel in his pocket, opened Penny's door, and got her out of the car. He glanced at the packages on the floor.

'I see you've bought a lot of vegetables from the market. Vegetable soup tonight?'

'Yes, if I have time to make it from scratch. You were back early today.'

'Mother and I had an argument, so I took her home early.' He held Penny firmly as he opened the front door.

'Yes, I know,' I said absently as I concentrated on getting the vegetables out of the car quickly enough so that I could catch Penny before she started making too much of a fuss.

'Oh?' John looked at me. 'How do you know?' He went inside quickly, sat Penny in her playpen and turned to face me.

My cheeks felt very hot. 'I went to shop in Ely and I saw you and your mother in the distance.'

'That's strange; we were only there for a very short time. You must have been very close. Where were you?

'I popped into the Lamb Hotel for a coffee.'

'What, on your own?'

I grimaced. 'No.' I turned my back as I took the vegetables into the kitchen and put them on the sink.

'So who were you with?' John shouted making sure I could hear him.

'Oh,' I had run out of ideas. He would have to know sometime. 'Well, if you must know, Aunt Hannah and I had coffee together.'

'So!' he snapped, grabbed his package and stormed upstairs to his office. The door slammed.

Penny's mouth screwed up and she started wailing. I sighed, picked her up and cuddled her. 'Never mind, little one,' I murmured, 'the truth will out eventually.'

That evening, after I had managed to persuade Penny to go to sleep in her cot upstairs, I paused outside John's office door. I knocked gently. At dinner we had not mentioned my time with Hannah and had eased ourselves into a mundane conversation about other matters. It would be nice if we could heal the wounds by sitting down together and talking. We had not done that for a long time.

'Come in!' he said. I opened the door and walked in. His office was as pristine as ever, every file and piece of paper in its place. The phone directories were still standing to attention in their neat row on the bottom of the bookshelves. Even his pens and pencils were in a neat line on his desk. The only disorder was the loosely wrapped parcel in front of him.

'Hi,' he smiled. My heart missed a beat. I could never resist his boyish smile. 'Oh, yes,' he turned towards me, 'I forgot to ask, but I remember some time ago you said you were going to the library in Ely to look up which evening class you were going to take. Have you decided which one you would like to do?'

'I couldn't make up my mind so I've left it for a while,' I blushed. I hated telling lies. 'Besides,' I continued hurriedly, 'I'm not sure we can afford for me to do any more classes for a while. We should be paying off our debts and then saving.'

'I don't know what for,' said John, un-wrapping his parcel completely.

'Remember we agreed that we would look for a bigger house after we were settled?'

'Oh, that'll not be for ages yet.' John picked up the contents of his parcel. It was a silver plaque with the words 'Queen Elizabeth II Silver Jubilee 1977' engraved on it. 'What do you think of it? Won't Mother be pleased?'

'But I thought your mother's birthday was not for a good four months yet?'

'That's true, but she needs something to cheer her up now. I'll take it to her tomorrow.'

'How much did it cost? Where did you get the money from?'

'Just a few hundred pounds from our joint account.'

'A *few hundred pounds*!' I shouted.John looked at me as if I were being totally unreasonable. I was too shocked to say any more.

'I'll just check on Penny,' I murmured, scuttling rapidly out of the room before I said anything I regretted. As I looked at our sleeping baby, I decided that when I met the bank manager next Thursday I would definitely open a separate bank account.

Bliss! It was sheer bliss. After a month of waiting, I had finally been called to do some supply teaching at a local school. Babs was between jobs and had agreed to look after Penny and I was sitting in the busy staff room clutching a cup of coffee. Nothing would make me put it down, I did not have to stop my crawling baby from smashing a vase, someone else was answering the phone and there was no John asking me to take part in a newly contrived scheme.

'I've got to plan a syllabus.' Steve, my head of department, sat down next to me. I grimaced. Was this the interruption? Was I going to have to do this?

'It's all right,' he said, reading my expression exactly. 'I'll do it. I just wondered if you had any ideas about something you would like to have included.'

'No, whatever you say should be fine. I'm only on part-time supply anyway so you're the one who will have to put up with doing most of what you have decided.' I took another sip of coffee. Bliss.

'That's fine,' he said standing up. 'See you later.'

The bell for the next lesson rang. This time I was actually looking forward to teaching a classroom full of hormonally charged teenagers. It was so different after having a baby. Nothing seemed difficult after that.

'You know,' John said to me as I walked past his office to change Penny's cot, 'your dad's flight is so early in the morning next Wednesday, that I'll go and meet him and drive him to Peterborough. You can stay and look after Penny.'

My face fell. 'But I thought he would be staying with us or at least near here?'

'Oh no, Mother has arranged for him to stay at the Bull in Peterborough. He will be much more comfortable there.' He stood up, took his jacket off the back of his chair and smiled. 'I'll drive you to Peterborough with Penny to see him at the weekend.' He put his jacket on and walked purposefully out of his office. 'I'll just nip over to see Sam for a moment.' He stepped quickly downstairs and straight out the door.

Holding the clean sheet in my hand I stared after him. How dare they! He was my father and I desperately wanted to see him. Penny squawked. I walked smartly towards her.

'Ah it's lovely to see you, Sally.' Dad hugged Penny and me as though he would never let us go. 'And Penny.' He stepped back to look at her. 'Isn't she gorgeous?' he said proudly. I put Penny into his arms. She gurgled and patted his cheek. He held her like a precious china vase. Penny smiled and Dad grinned like I had never seen him grin before.

'Are you hungry?' he asked me, while pulling a face at Penny. Penny giggled.

'Oh yes,' I said and we went towards the restaurant.

It was when we were having coffee that the trouble started.

'Your mother is a lovely lady,' Dad said to John. I choked on my coffee. 'Sorry,' I said between my bouts of spluttering. I wiped the coffee from my cheeks and chest. Penny banged her high chair. I quickly gave her my teaspoon.

'Yes,' said John reservedly. 'She has had a difficult time of it. I'll just pop to the bar and get some more sugar.' John stood up and left the table.

Dad leaned towards me. 'Sally,' he almost whispered. 'How would you feel if I asked Eunice to marry me?'

Chapter 21

I froze. I could not believe what I had heard. Surely Dad must know what my mother-in-law was really like? How could he even think of having anything to do with her? *Marriage*? He must be joking! But then, Dad is a man and has a man's blinkered vision of what a woman can truly be like. Would he really want to be harangued and nagged the way John is? Surely not! I ought to say I would be delighted, but I couldn't. I couldn't deceive my dad, a man without an evil bone in his body.

'Dad,' I said, looking him straight in his eyes, ignoring the noise that was coming from Penny's highchair. 'You don't know the half of it. Mother-in-law may not have shown you one of her tantrums yet, but believe me, you do *not* want a life of those. If you marry her,' I snarled, 'you'll get a miserable life that you don't deserve!' I grabbed the teaspoon from Penny who let out a loud wail.

Dad paled and looked down at the table.

'Trouble?' John asked as he sat down again.

'No,' Dad and I chorused. Penny looked up at her dad, her cheeks running with tears. My hands were trembling as I lifted her out of the highchair.

Dad left to go back to Tasmania. Mother-in-law was particularly difficult the next week but otherwise everything returned to normal. I decided to keep quiet about the rest of his family for the time being. As John was constantly saying; 'Anything for a quiet life.'

The school holidays soon came and John had arranged for us to stay with Bill and Mary on their pig farm. I was looking forward to seeing them again and was glad that there would be at least one good memory of my time with John to rekindle our relationship. I smiled as I thought of that afternoon in the lane near Bill and Mary's house when John had asked me to marry him. It seemed a lifetime ago.

Our journey was smooth and uneventful. Penny slept all the way and I was content to let John do the driving. As the smooth hills of the Essex countryside gradually appeared I could feel the tension in my shoulders relax.

Mary greeted us with drinks in the garden. I went off to feed and change Penny and when I went back outside, John and Bill had gone to busy themselves about the farm. Mary was sitting on a large rug, enjoying the late afternoon sunshine. I put Penny down next to her and before I could sit down she said, 'You go and rest a bit, I'll look after the baby.'

'Oh, thank you!' I cried. Mary did not know how grateful I was. I walked up their garden path, climbed up the stairs and flopped down on the bed for a rest.

'Thank you so much,' I said when, feeling much better, I found Mary in the kitchen. Penny was gurgling happily. 'How has she been?'

'She has been fine. I've given her a bath and changed her. I hope that was all right.'

'All right? That's wonderful. I'll look after her now.' I picked up Penny and laughed with her.

'I'm going to start the tea, if that's all right. You enjoy the last of the sun.'

I left Mary in the kitchen and went to sit down outside on the rug with Penny. The sun was still quite high. The trees were rustling in the breeze and dappled shadows darted across the lawn. A peacock screeched in a far-off field. Closer to hand the crows were squawking in the wood at the bottom of the garden. The air was fresh. There was no smell of the pigs this time as they were much further down the farm and the wind was being kind to us.

Suddenly, without warning, tears streamed down my cheeks. Why was I crying? I was fine — or was I? Hadn't I heard about the baby blues? Surely the blues did not happen as late as this? Penny looked up at me enquiringly as I let the tears flow. I hugged her. Some day she would understand.

Mary served a lovely full breakfast the next morning. After my first mouthful I dashed to the bathroom and promptly vomited.

'You must be allergic to mushrooms. Can I get you something else?' Mary offered.

'No, no it's fine. I don't think I am allergic to mushrooms — cooked tomatoes maybe — but not mushrooms.'

I knew I wasn't allergic to mushrooms. When we returned home I found out the cause of my sickness. I was pregnant.

'Pregnant?' John exclaimed. 'How did that happen?'

We were both surprised. I had been sure that we had never made love at the vital part of the month. The rhythm method was our method of contraception. Never again!

I grinned. 'Well, we always wanted another baby — not quite yet, maybe, but this will get it all over and done with in a few years. They say the first five years of a marriage are the busiest.'

John hugged me. He was going to be a father again!

'You know,' I said pulling away for a moment. 'We ought to move to a detached house. A semi-detached is no place for children.'

'It is in England.'

'Yes, but when I was a child in Tasmania nobody lived in a semi-detached house. Our neighbour bangs the wall when I play my scales on the piano, anyway. It would be lovely to be able to play the piano again without someone banging on the wall.'

'Maybe.' John was thinking.

'And remember when the neighbour's teenager decided to shoot his rifle within a few feet of the baby? It would be lovely if we could feel safe and the children could play.'

'I'll think about it.' John grabbed his coat. 'I'll just pop over to Mother's. I'll ask her what she thinks.' I grimaced as his car pulled out of the driveway.

I checked that Penny was happily playing and quickly dashed upstairs to search our joint bank account statements. Yes, the manager had done his bit and we had not overspent. Although John had complained about the bank manager, he had not yet realized that I had arranged the curtailment of his spending. I dashed downstairs and searched the drawer in the desk downstairs and looked at my account. Yes, we had managed to pay off most of our debts and now was definitely the time to move.

'John,' I said over breakfast the following Friday morning, 'We won't move until you're happy.' The detached house issue was becoming a bit repetitive. 'But look, here is a place in Witchford. It's only in the next village. It's within our price range.' I pushed the papers towards him.

'I'll look into it tonight,' he said, taking a last bite of his toast. 'Has it got all the utility bills, how much everything would cost?'

'Yes, I asked the estate agent to include them all.'

'All right, then. I'll look into it, but no promises.'

'No, we won't do anything until you're happy.' I stared at him, my unswerving eyes daring him to disagree.

'Be careful!' I called as the removal men staggered through the snow. The huge box they were carrying teetered to their right. They swung it back into line and struggled towards the open front door. 'It's a blue box so it's for the dining room. Please remember to stick to the colour code.'

I was cold, my bump was only just obvious and the move was taking ages. I looked at the garden of our new house. It was beautiful. Daffodils stretched to the other end of the large plot that went with the detached house.

'It's like staying in a luxurious hotel,' I said to John as we lay in our new bed that evening. 'And it's all ours.'

'It's going to cost us a lot more.'

'I know, but we agreed. We're mortgaged up to the hilt, but we can do it. If the worst happens, I could go out to work full time.'

'No, no. It won't come to that.' John kissed me.

'Penny will be one year old next month. Imagine that!' I mused. John kissed me again. 'We'll have to have a party.'

'That would be lovely,' he murmured.

The week of the party arrived.

'Mother isn't coming,' John said as he came in the door, late from work again.

'Why not?'

'She says you're jealous of her.' He hung up his coat. 'Why are you jealous?'

'Jealous? *Me*? I'm *not* jealous of her.' I slammed down the knife I was drying into the drawer. 'Why won't she come to our daughter's birthday party? Is it because the party is not for her?'

'That's beside the point. The point is why don't you treat her like your own mother?'

I saw red. 'You want me to treat her like my own mother? Give me the phone book.' I rattled through the pages until I found the number. With trembling fingers I dialled.

'Hello,' the voice was graceful, smooth.

'It's Sally here. Why won't you come to our Penny's birthday party?'

There was a moment of silence.

'I would not enjoy it.'

'Look, it wouldn't hurt you to come for just a few minutes. We'll do everything you want. We'll look after you.'

The voice was silent. The phone line went dead. Just as I was leaving the room, the phone rang again.

'Ah, she's changed her mind,' I called to John. But the voice was not my mother-in-law's. It was another woman's voice, an unfamiliar one.

'I am a close friend of Eunice,' the voice said. 'You have always created trouble for this family. I hated you from the moment I saw you. I am going to do all I can to split you two up. I hope your baby dies.' The voice was unmoved, cold, calculating. I managed a maniacal laugh and put the phone down.

'John?' He stared. 'A friend of your mother's.'

'Oh?'

'She said she hoped our baby dies.'

'Mm.' He paled.

'Haven't you got any more to say about it?' John walked slowly out of the house to his car.

The birthday party was messy and noisy, but fun. Mother-in-law did not come.

John started coming home from work earlier and earlier each day. He obviously wasn't calling at his mother's. Then he worked more and more at home, into the late evening.

'Have you been seeing all the customers you should?' I asked. There was something amiss with his work, I could tell.

'No, I see all my customers and after that I've got to see how Mother is, so I stop at hers for a while. Anyway, I've got a lot of paperwork to do. Are you going to get me a cup of tea?' I put the kettle on, checked Penny was not into mischief in the playroom and set out the cups and saucers.

John sighed and looked into his teacup. 'I think I had better get another job, with the new baby coming and all.' He frowned, his hands were shaking. He was tense. How could I stop him feeling so tense?

'No you don't, we'll manage,' I said, sitting next to him, keeping an ear out for the toddler.

'Well, I've been putting in applications and I have got an interview at Oakham tomorrow.'

'An interview? So soon?' I hugged him. His shoulders were tight. 'Well done! You must be doing well to get an interview. Good luck.' I thought nothing more of it.

The next day I stolidly went through the routine. As the hours ticked by and the early afternoon beckoned, I was looking forward to the time when Penny and I would have our afternoon nap. Just before then the phone rang.

'Hello?' I asked, trying to lift my voice above the chortles of the toddler nearby.

'It's John.'

'You sound distant.'

'I'm ringing from a call box. I'm about to go into the hotel for my interview.'

'Well, good luck. I'll keep my fingers crossed. You can do it.'

'Bye' he said, sounding cool and aloof, as if this were some kind of farewell call. I shrugged my shoulders. I felt flattered that he needed some words of good luck and confidence-boosting praise before he went into an interview. But why did he sound so distracted?

You would expect him to be trying to be really focused on his job. Penny started to get irritable with her toys. At last she was tired and we could both have a rest. The new baby was growing more and more, and the more it grew, the more I was desperate for my afternoon rest. My eyelids were dropping at the thought of it. I stretched out on the bed and closed my eyes. Bliss.

The phone jangled. How could anyone phone now of all times!

'Hello?' I said slowly, my eyes not fully focused.

'Is that Mrs Wilks?'

'Yes.'

'This is the nurse at Peterborough Hospital. We have your husband here.'

I sat up. 'But he's in Oakham. He's having an interview at Oakham.' I swung round and let my feet touch the floor. 'Is there something wrong? Is he conscious?'

'He's in Ward Six if you would like to see him.'

Why hadn't she answered my question? *Was* he conscious or would she not say because he wasn't? I stood in the centre of the room. What was I to do? I went out to the landing, pacing up and down. What could I do? I couldn't just drive there. I had been told I had to have another caesarean. What if I went into shock with this news? I dithered.

I rushed outside. I needed someone to help me. I rushed to Mildred Thomas's door. Mildred would see me through this. She had stopped me in the street so many times and had wanted to know all about us. She would love to be involved. The rose rambling over her doorway was in its last stages of blooming for the summer. I pushed the doorbell and banged on her door loudly. The house was silent. Why doesn't she answer the door? She was always in. Then I remembered, today was her shopping day, the one day in the week when she went to town. I muttered under my breath and went immediately to the house between hers and ours.

I did not really want to rouse Leonie. She was always so distant, quite uninvolved in village business. The door swung open. Leonie looked at me glumly.

Chapter 22

'Yes?' Leonie held onto the door rigidly.

'Leonie, I'm so glad to have caught you in,' I panted. 'I'm sorry to disturb you but John is in hospital. Can you come over to my house and supervise me while I make phone calls? I'm not sure how I will cope. I might go into shock.'

Leonie paused looking through me as though she were weighing up a situation that had nothing to do with the explanation I had given. We had never been really close. I found Leonie and her husband to be the sort of people who keep up with the Joneses at all costs. This did not match well with my easy-going casual style of neighbourliness and housekeeping. I remembered how Leonie could not quite conceal her nose twitching with displeasure at the creative chaos that was my sitting room when she had come in for her first and last coffee. But now it was different, it was an emergency and I could not believe that anyone could refuse to help. After all, I was only asking her to supervise a few phone calls. She reluctantly followed me into our house. She looked straight ahead, avoiding the chaos that Penny had left before I had taken her upstairs to sleep. Leonie stood still and watched me while I phoned Babs to care for Penny, and Aunty Janice to be next to John's bed quickly so that he could recognize her when or if he became conscious again and finally Paul Saunders, a kind neighbour several doors away on the other side to Leonie and recently retired, who would drive me to the hospital in case I went into labour and we had to retrace our steps and go to Cambridge Hospital.

When I entered the ward John was vomiting into a bowl, flopping back on his pillows and passing back into unconsciousness. He had a large black eye.

'Oh, John,' I cried as I rushed to his side. 'Thank you,' I said quickly to Aunty Janice who was sitting next to him.

She gave me a hug, 'I'm so sorry. If there is anything I can do...'

I hugged her back as tears welled up in my eyes. She knew that my throat was too constricted to reply. She hugged me again and said, 'When he first awoke he asked me if you had farrowed yet.' She smiled. I returned her smile weakly. Some of the old John was still there! In vain had I tried to persuade him to stop likening me to a farm animal — 'I am not a pig!' I had retorted each time he likened me to one. John sat up, vomited and flopped down again.

I sat down on the chair next to the bed, waved goodbye to Aunty Janice and wondered if it would be better to try to wake John properly, or to leave him so that he didn't have to be sick so many times. I decided to wait for the moment.

'This is really very inconvenient,' a strong voice echoed in the corridor. A chill ran up my spine. I could recognize that voice anywhere. It was my mother-in-law!

'This is very thoughtless of you,' she said towards the body in the bed that was her son. 'I had so many other things to do today, and the last thing I wanted was to come and see you here in this state.' John sat up to vomit.

I pushed the bump forwards between John and his mother and said quickly before John fell back again,

'Do you want us to talk or do you want peace?'

'Peace,' he whimpered and sank into unconsciousness.

His mother stood open-mouthed, glared at me and then at John and hurried away to speak to the nurses.

Later that afternoon I picked up the phone.

'Aunty Janice?'

'You know you said if there was anything else you could do?

'Yes, anything dear. You know that.'

'Well,' I bit my lip. 'My daughter and I need to be in Peterborough near John. Can you help out?'

'Of course we can.' Her voice was calm and sympathetic. Tears sprang in my eyes.

I gulped before speaking again. 'I know Uncle Tom doesn't like children. Will he really be all right with my toddler in his house?'

'Of course he will. Don't you worry about that. We'll see you in a few hours. I'll make the beds up for you.'

The tears were streaming down my face as I packed and Paul drove me to Uncle Tom's.

On the first return visit to the hospital, I walked into John's ward. He was still in bed. He was now more conscious but he stared at me as though I were a stranger, this man I knew intimately, this man whose whole body had been explored by my searching fingers, this man whose complex personality I had come to understand. This was my husband, father of Penny and an integral part of our lives and yet he looked at me as if he had never seen me before. I shuddered.

'He has had some kind of accident.' The doctor sat next to me. 'People can lose their memories when this happens.' The doctor was using his best bedside comforting tone. I raised my eyebrows.

'Sometimes the memory returns suddenly, sometimes it comes back very slowly, bit by bit. If you can remind him of his past and his current life this should help jolt his memory a lot.'

I sat next to John and held his hand. He looked startled for a moment. One of John's colleagues swept onto the ward.

'Hello, John.' John stared at him, his eyes flickering in a brief moment of recognition.

'Sorry to see you in such a state and sorry to trouble you, but do you know where you parked the car?'

'Oakham,' John mumbled, sounding as if he were responding automatically, as though there was no real meaning behind it.

'Oh,' I butted in, 'he was going for an interview in Oakham. He went to a hotel there. I think his keys are in his jacket pocket.' I lifted my bulk out of the chair, went to his jacket and extricated the keys.

'Thank you, I'm sure we'll find it. Don't you worry, John. I'll see to everything.'

John stared at his colleague.

I sat down heavily. 'Well, John, in case you don't remember, I'm your wife and the bump I'm carrying is your second child. Our daughter Penny is with your Uncle Tom and Aunty Janice.' He stared.

'You've got a tremendous black eye,' I said.

'What black eye?' He was interested.

I got a mirror out of my purse and held it up to him so he could see it.

'I wonder how you got that?' I asked with a faint smile. 'Fighting again, eh?'

He looked blank.

In the evening, I returned to the haven of Aunty Janice and Uncle Tom's place. Penny ran to meet me and I picked her up and went to the kitchen. I put Penny down on the floor and she moved towards Uncle Tom and played with his shoelaces.

'You know,' said Uncle Tom, smiling down at Penny, 'you can stay here as long as you like. I like having you both here.' I looked at Aunty Janice, who winked.

'He really means it!' she said.

'It's a pity Eunice is so difficult,' Uncle Tom murmured, taking down three glasses from the cupboard. 'She's my sister, but I can't help wondering if she might have had more to do with Walter's brother's problems than she would let on.'

'I know, dear.' Aunty Janice reached up for a plastic cup for Penny. 'A friend of mine used to work at Matthew's car firm.' She looked at Tom sideways, as if weighing up what to say next. He sat on the stool at the kitchen bar and looked at her, his face smooth and untroubled.

She filled Penny's cup with juice, put the lid on and handed it to Penny, who snatched it and drank thirstily. 'Only last week when we were having coffee, she said she saw Eunice in the office several times before Matthew was accused of stealing.'

'They were going out together then, weren't they?' Uncle Tom filled our glasses with wine.

Aunty Janice took her glass and put it down on the bar, sitting on the stool next to her husband. I joined them. Penny banged her empty cup on the floor rhythmically.

'Yes,' said Aunty Janice. 'Cheers — here's to the next great niece or great nephew, eh?' We chinked glasses. Aunty Janice continued, 'One day when she was going towards the office she saw Eunice through the window quickly screwing up a piece of paper and throwing it in the bin. When she went into the office, Eunice looked so guilty that she wondered what she had been up to. She waited until Eunice and Matthew had left and she found the scrap of paper. It contained a number of Matthew's signatures as though Eunice had been trying to forge them. Just as she was about to put the piece of paper in her pocket, Eunice came back and snatched it from her.'

'Why didn't she say something to the authorities about this at the time?' Uncle Tom asked.

'She says she did. She says she told Matthew but he would not listen and the police said there was no real evidence. It had been destroyed.' We sat subdued. Penny's banging was louder and more insistent.

'Come on little one,' Aunty Janice said, and lifted Penny into the highchair. 'I'll get you something to eat.'

Day after day I chatted to John. Little by little he came back to me. It was heart breaking but after five days, I was certain that John recognized me at last. His memory was returning.

A brisk nurse brought in clean bedding. She turned to me and said, 'He's ready to go home now. You can take him home tomorrow.'

'But what happened? What was wrong with him?'

'We're not sure.'

'But you must know. I can't take him home without knowing what was wrong with him,' I said anxiously.

The nurse hurried towards the door. 'I'm very sorry, but we may never know. The doctor says that he's all right now and that's what matters.' She left.

So John, his black eye still visible, his mind still slightly confused, came home. He sat in his chair in the sitting room watching as the toddler and I went on with our daily lives.

I went to Cambridge Hospital for my usual check-up.

'My husband was found unconscious in the street at Oakham and he has only just returned home,' I reported to the doctor.

'When is the baby due? Ah, I see it's only two weeks away,' the doctor said as he scanned the chart. 'I think we'd better schedule a caesarean for tomorrow. We'll know where we are then.'

'Tomorrow?' I gulped. 'But -' Flashes of the horror of my last caesarean crashed into my thoughts. I wasn't ready. But what if the baby started coming and I was at home? It would be more sensible to get it over and done with now. I looked at the doctor. He looked calm and reassuring.

I said softly, 'All right then, tomorrow.' I was resigned to my fate. I rushed out as fast as my huge frame would allow, drove home and started making arrangements.

Chapter 23

At home, John sat in his chair, still numb from his experience in hospital. Penny happily climbed over the sofa, strangled the draught excluder and rearranged the cushions on the chairs. John hardly noticed as I rushed up and down the stairs preparing the cot, the pram and the nappies for the arrival of the new baby, phoning down the list of friends to help take care of Penny and warning people I would be out of circulation for a while.

'I'll drive you in,' John mumbled, unconvincingly. My heart sank. He did not realize he would not be able to drive again, not for two years at least.

'It's all right, John.' I tried to sound as though the information I was about to give was not very important, just an afterthought. 'Remember, you're not allowed to drive again until the doctor says you can.' I paused mid-flight across the sitting room to look at my husband.

He grunted scathingly.

I continued, 'Paul will drive me in and he says he'll bring you and Penny in for visits. All right?'

John mumbled, 'I suppose so.'

I was left on my own on the hospital bed, my large bump preventing me from seeing the woman opposite, who had recently given birth. Perhaps it was for the best. The searing pain of the knife that sliced me open while I was still awake last time returned to me in a blinding flash. No, not again, I couldn't go through that again. But I had no choice. I patted my bump. The baby had to come out somehow. Was I ready for days without sleep, hourly feeds, and a baby that never settled? I sighed. I didn't feel ready but there was no choice.

Two gowned figures approached my bed.

'We've come to take you to the operating theatre.' One of them adjusted my bed and they started wheeling it out of the ward.

I panicked. I shrieked. 'No, no, I've changed my mind' I tried to joke, but they all knew this was no joke. This was real terror. 'The last time I was still awake when they cut me open. Please, please make sure I'm properly unconscious this time!' My voice rose with each new utterance. 'No! No! I can't have the baby anyway, I haven't thought of a name!' I screamed as they approached the theatre doors.

A nurse stood beside the bed, patted my hand and stayed with me until I swallowed something, and a horrible taste filled the back of my mouth. I finally succumbed to the all-embracing blackness of unconsciousness.

I woke back in the ward. Pain. Where was the pain? There was NO pain! Fantastic! I could do this again, I thought. My wound was strapped so tightly that I could sit up without feeling I was going to split apart. Wonderful! Wonderful!

A nurse placed a bundle carefully into my arms, saying, 'You have a lovely girl, seven pounds and all is well.'

I looked at the little face, felt the little fingers and grinned. 'She's beautiful. How could I have thought she was going to be a boy?' I thought of a name. 'She's going to be Emma.'

I fed Emma easily, put her in the cot beside my bed to sleep and settled down for a snooze myself. I was woken by the loud clatter of a toddler's feet on the linoleum floor of the ward. I would know those little feet anywhere. It was Penny! I felt a thump on my wound. Penny had climbed onto her Mum's bed.

'Mummy!' I looked into my daughter's shining smile framed by a bunch of red curls. John stood next to the bed beaming, his hands holding a bunch of flowers awkwardly, his eyes filled with tears.

'I had to be brought here by Paul.' He stood as if waiting to be told what to do. I lifted myself into an upright position and leaned over carefully to pick up the baby.

I said to John, 'Would you like to hold her?'

He put the flowers on my bedside table and held his arms out. Penny climbed off the bed and grabbed her dad's jacket as she strained to see.

I said quickly, 'Don't forget to support her head.' John held the baby self-consciously. He could not stop the tears flowing.

Penny patted her dad's jacket. 'No cry, Daddy,' she said.

John put the baby carefully into my arms, took out a handkerchief from his pocket and wiped his eyes. I noticed the handkerchief had not been washed for some time.

I let him finish wiping his eyes, and put on my motherly voice. 'I'll be going to the Grange in Ely to convalesce and to let the baby settle into a routine.' I tried to keep the unease out of my voice. 'You'll be all right, won't you? If you have any problems, just call Babs.'

John grinned. 'While the cat's away, the mice will play. I'll look after Penny. Everything will be fine. After all the neighbours are queuing up to feed us.'

I smiled. 'You'd better go and catch up with Penny; she seems to be leaving the ward already.'

John turned and ran to catch up with the little figure that was staring at a family next to the open doors to the ward.

I fell back onto the bed. I was exhausted. I would not worry about what was going on at home. John and Penny would just have to cope.

Emma and I were taken by taxi to the nursing home in Ely. It was magnificent. It was in a large campus, the spotless white buildings surrounded by fields and mature trees. It was the Royal Air Force Hospital built to see that the members of the Royal Air Force and their family were treated well. I was the only patient and the nurses were delighted to have someone to care for. I was in a large room that overlooked huge chestnut trees. I stared out of the window. In a moment I was transported back in time. It was as if I were one of the many air force wives nurtured by a caring community that looked after the families of the treasured air corps during the war.

The nurses brought the baby to me when she wanted a feed. I kicked off my slippers and slid onto the bed. I suddenly felt alone. My future looked uncertain: a baby, a toddler, an awkward husband who had just recovered from some kind of accident and a troublesome mother-in-law. I felt weighed down by insurmountable pressures. I looked at the photo of Penny on the table next to me. The smiling redheaded child in the picture looked at me quizzically. I was overwhelmed with love, pure love. At that moment I realized that I adored this child and we had created such a bond that it enveloped me entirely. I was not alone. There was someone who loved me, really loved me. This was not to say that John did not love me — for it is certain that he did, but in his own unique way. But I learnt in this moment that there is such as thing as 'motherly love'. I lay back in the pillows, smiling, and dozed.

The taxi finally pulled up outside our home.

'Ah! Sally's home,' Mildred Thomas, the granny figure from two doors down, who had decided to take us under her wing once she heard about John's accident, rushed towards the car. 'Can I see? Can I see?' Mildred opened the car door for me. I levered myself out carefully, clutching the baby close to me and making sure I did not hit the side of the car doorway as I stepped out.

'She's beautiful,' Mildred cooed.

I glowed. 'Yes, she is, isn't she?'

The front door of the house was flung open. 'Mummy, mummy!' Penny rushed out and clutched my legs.

'We must go inside,' I said to Mildred, as I walked carefully towards the open door, Penny still clutching my skirt.

John eventually came forward.

'Thank goodness you've come home!' he said with real feeling.

'Has everything been all right?' I asked as I went into the sitting room with Emma and Penny.

'Well, Babs and the choirgirls have helped a bit. There was one night I really couldn't get Penny changed,' John slumped quickly in his chair. 'I phoned up Sarah and one of the girls came round to help.'

'Thank goodness your company has been so understanding. Will you be going back to work on Monday?'

'No,' John snapped. The tension in the room mounted. Emma squirmed. She needed feeding. Penny was stroking Emma's blanket.

I gritted my teeth. 'Why not?'

'I'm on permanent sick leave.'

'Permanent?'

John looked down at the floor.

I lifted Emma over my shoulder, stood up and rocked her a little. Penny sucked her thumb and sulked. Her baby sister had been taken away from her.

I asked, 'Surely it's for a period of six months or so and then you return to your work?'

'No, I have sick pay for a while and then they want me to leave.' He shifted his feet on the carpet that was sorely in need of vacuuming.

'Oh, John, I am sorry,' I tried to sound sympathetic but myriad thoughts crowded into my mind. If he was going to be unemployed what were we to do? Where would the money come from? I was not ready for work. I went pale, clutched Emma more closely and went upstairs to change and feed her.

The days and nights passed quickly in a flow of never-ending nightmares and energy-sapping activity, looking after two very young children and worrying about the future. John's months of sickness would run out soon and he was not ready to return to his job. He sat in his chair day after day hardly moving. It was as if he were a tall, sturdy tree that had had all the sap drained out. He was lethargic, not lazy, just empty and unable to do anything, as though he were in deep shock.

Like an automated zombie I allowed myself to be caught up in the exhausting rituals. I ran up and down the stairs, chasing after the toddler, serving John's needs, giving him meals that he did not enjoy and feeding and looking after baby Emma. My dresses started fitting me better. I must have been losing weight! At least there was something positive about my frantic life at the moment.

Every night baby Emma seemed unhappy after her last feed when I put her down to sleep. I did not understand it. The baby was clean, dry and she had been fed. I continued in the ritual — what else could I do?

'I don't know what to do, John,' I sat in the sitting room holding the weeping baby close. 'She doesn't seem right.'

'What am I supposed to do about it?' John snapped. My heart went cold. I was never going to get any sympathy here. Life could be so cruel.

'Your baby is not gaining weight,' the young health visitor looked earnestly into my eyes. My shoulders drooped. I looked back at her in puzzlement.

'I think you should take her to hospital for a short while until her feeding pattern becomes more established.'

Hospital? Surely things were not as drastic as that! What would happen to John and Penny? I sighed looking down at my feet. I had failed. But I would have some time alone with Emma, maybe even time to get some rest. No running after or battling with John, a complete day's rest. I smiled weakly and nodded.

I lay back on the hospital bed. The bustling noise of other people, nurses and trolleys banging against the beds were a welcome background hum. Rest at last. Emma was asleep next to me. I dozed.

'It's time for her feed,' the nurse handed me a warm bottle of milk for Emma. This was the first time she would not be breast-fed. How would she take it?

I held Emma in my arms and placed the teat of the bottle onto her lips. Emma closed her lips tight. I touched them again. She would not budge. It was a battle of wills and if I did not win little Emma would not thrive. I looked around the ward despairingly. It was a matter of life and death. I *had* to win. I gripped the baby firmly and touched her lips with the teat of the bottle again. The lips remained firmly shut. Weeping, I tried a third time and nothing happened. I pursed my lips, took a deep breath and made a fourth attempt, pushing the bottle hard onto the baby's lips. She still kept them firmly closed. I let out a cry of despair.

'You *will* take the bottle!' I shouted, pushing harder, willing the child to open her lips and let the life-giving milk flow into her mouth. Emma's lips parted a fraction. My hands shaking, I pushed the bottle hard into the tiny gap and Emma's mouth opened just enough and closed round the teat. She sucked. At last! Tears of joy slid down my flushed cheeks.

The taxi pulled up at our house. The front door opened. John stepped forward looking tired and irritable.

'You're home at last then.' He stood in front of the door, unaware that he was blocking my entrance to the house.

'Can you move aside a bit so that I can get in?' I asked, baby Emma on one arm and my case held by the other. He finally moved aside as I struggled into the house.

'It's been really hard while you've been away.' He closed the door and followed me upstairs as I dumped the case in our bedroom, grabbed a sheet from the airing cupboard and placed the sleeping Emma in her cot.

'Has Penny been?' I asked. 'Where is she?'

'She's at Sarah's,' John said. 'I couldn't get Penny dressed this morning, so I rang Sarah and she said she would look after her for a bit.'

'The Reverend David Halls called,' John said as he followed me downstairs into the kitchen where I started preparing Emma's bottles. 'He would be pleased to baptize Emma.'

'Jolly good,' I murmured, as I made sure I was measuring the sterilizing agent accurately.

'He said he could do it on the 5th of November, Guy Fawkes Day.'

'Okay.' I went into the sitting room to find my purse and the diary in it. I took out the diary and wrote in the date.

'What time?' I asked John, who was standing in the sitting room doorway.

'He was a student in Cambridge. He has baptized over fifty babies, you know.'

'What time is the baptism?' I repeated.

John looked at me blankly. 'Eleven o'clock. All the godparents will have to be there. They will have to promise to see that Emma goes to church and obeys the church rules.'

'I need to check on Emma, she will need changing and feeding again soon.' I went towards the sitting room door. John was still standing in the doorway blocking my exit. I looked at him. He did not move. I could hear Emma crying upstairs.

'For goodness sake,' I shouted. 'Will you move out of the way?'

John slowly stepped away from the door into the hall. He looked at me, hurt and puzzled. I pushed against him as I ran upstairs.

Chapter 24

I turned the page. I was tired but not too tired to wonder whodunit. I was too lazy to try to work it out for myself but the book was well written. I could enjoy the characters' interactions and their conversations. John and I were relaxing in bed after an arduous day. The children's rooms were silent. I would soon unwind and be able to drift off into much-needed sleep.

Suddenly John cried out. I turned swiftly to see why. His face was contorted; his eyes were open and rolling back into his head. Was he suddenly dying? What was happening? His whole body shook and his legs and arms jerked wildly.

'John!' I cried, but he could not hear me. I held his shoulders but they shook beneath my hands as if I were not even there. It was as if a malevolent being had struck him, got inside his brain and was playing havoc with the electrical circuit. I sat back, helpless, watching while his body contorted in a maniacal way. I moved to touch him, but he was oblivious to my presence. What could I do? How could I help him?

Then I realized. He was having an epileptic fit! Open-mouthed, heart pounding, I stared at my husband's writhing body. If I were superstitious, I thought, it could be easy to imagine that he was being possessed, that he was being infected with a mysterious evil spirit that was claiming him as part of a dark world of malicious spells and witchcraft.

I shook my head, forced myself to overcome the horror of what was happening. It was just an epileptic fit. I'm a teacher, I reminded myself. I know about these things. I can cope. In the back of my mind stirred a thought. There was something about stopping him from swallowing his tongue, wasn't there? I pushed my book towards his mouth. It was impossible. His teeth were clenched far too tight. I lay back, inert, helpless, watching his reddened face, his shaking limbs. His body was so rigid. I was so helpless.

At last his limbs stopped jerking. He lay on his back, still. Then he slowly turned on his side. He would sleep now. His body would calm down and readjust so that when he woke in the morning he would be better. I sighed with relief.

But he did not sleep. He sat up.

'John?' I said. 'What are you doing? John?' I put my hand on his back as if to wake him from this terrible trance but there was no response. He stood up and in uncertain steps but with his own brand of determination he stepped through the open door and onto the landing. The stairs! I never knew someone could move about while still in a fit. He could fall down the stairs!

I threw my book on the floor, dashed outside the room and slipped behind him. I rushed to the fire door at the top of the stairs and shut it quickly. John had turned and was moving towards the bathroom door.

'John? John?' I cried again. There was no response. His hands were close to the bathroom door handle. This was too much for me. I couldn't cope.

I dashed back to our room, grabbed the phone and dialled.

'Hello?'

'Dad! Dad!' I shrieked. The words tumbled out of my mouth. 'John's just had an epileptic fit and he's moving about the house. I can't control him. He could fall down the stairs. He could shut himself in the bathroom and not be able to get out. I don't know what to do!'

'Sally,' said my father's voice. Oh how wonderful it was to hear the voice of my father, a friendly voice from someone who knew me and loved me, someone I could turn to in a crisis. The fact that he was in Australia, on the opposite side of the world, didn't make any difference. It was my father. He would help me.

There was a pause on the phone.

'You know,' his words were very carefully placed. 'I think you will have to rely on the doctors. Ask their advice. They will help you.'

'Yes, yes, the doctor,' I mumbled. 'Gee, thanks, Dad.' I smashed the receiver down, grabbed the phone book and finally dialled the doctor's number.

Two years passed and John was still a traumatized figure who could do no more than declare the contents of the newspaper. He was unaware of most of the events that happened around him but he was insistent that I and anyone else who was in earshot should understand what was happening in the world according to the newspapers he was avidly reading. Something had to happen. Keeping an ear out for the children crashing about in the playroom at the back of the house, I waved our joint bank statement, the one we were supposed to live on, in front of John and said:

'Look, we are not making ends meet. You've got to do something.'

'What am I supposed to do?' he snarled back. 'They've taken away my licence. I can't drive.'

'Well, you've got to *do* something; you can't live in your own depressive world much longer. You've got to get some money from somewhere. In two months' time we won't be able to pay the mortgage.' I had not told him that even though I had opened my own account, I had been unable to save anything since we had bought the new house.

John looked sullenly at the floor.

I moved to stand directly in front of him. 'You've got to borrow some money from your uncle. He will be able to tell you what to do too.'

John did not reply. He stood up slowly and went upstairs to his office. With my hands on my hips, I watched him go. I was surprised he was going to do it. I thought it would stir him into action and that he would try to get another job, not swallow all his pride and ask Uncle Tom for a loan. He really was at rock bottom.

John remained unemployed and his Uncle Tom paid the mortgage that month.

'Something's got to happen,' I shared with my choir friends. 'I've worked out if we don't do something soon we won't be able to pay the mortgage next month.'

'Ooh, that's terrible,' said Sharon, an architect's wife. 'It's awful when people lose their house. The men coming to claim it back are so horrible. They come into the house and throw everything outside. It doesn't bear thinking about.'

'No, it doesn't bear thinking about,' I agreed, my chin jutting out.

After the choir ladies left, I sat down alone. I had to do something. I could be John's carer and we could go on benefits. But I could not see myself as one of society's spongers, one of the down-and-outs who needed handouts. I could not bear the thought of it. Besides, I had had so much trouble with bureaucracy about getting the Child Benefit money due to us — did I want any more trouble like that? No, definitely not. The face of one particular bossy bureaucrat, who had kept saying she had our interests at heart, flashed into my thoughts. Harriet Bendall, with her straitjacketed personality, tight-lipped platitudes and ineffectiveness, was the last thing I wanted. But if I did nothing, I knew I would sink into the same depths of despair that John now lived in. What would be the point of that? No, I was going to beat this. I was not going to sink down to John's level. I was not going to have our lives made wretched by a lot of harrowing visits by Harriet Bendall 'helping' us fill in piles of forms. Besides, staying at home had never worked for me before. I needed to get out, *do* something. There was no question; I would go out to work. It was half term next week. I had one week to find work and a child-minder for the children. John could not cope; that was now clear.

The next few days were busier than I had ever known. I found a job starting the next Monday and, by a stroke of luck, I found a child minder a few miles away who would take my babies on that Monday morning. I employed a plump, non-nonsense cleaning lady, Mrs Brown, suggested by Babs, and crossed my fingers, hoping we would survive.

Tears welled up in my eyes as I watched my two toddlers, hand in hand tottering up to the child minder's door. They were both in nappies. It was too cruel.

Days and nights of utter exhaustion followed.

Late one Wednesday night I lay in bed, too exhausted to sleep. I sighed. At least it was the holidays and it did not matter if I did not sleep. John was in his office poring over his papers. I crawled out of bed, put on my dressing gown and slippers and stumbled towards the office.

'It's late, John,' I whispered so that I did not wake up the girls, 'come to bed.'

'I'll be there in a minute,' he snarled.

I looked over his shoulder. He was staring at a letter from the bank. The manager demanded an appointment to see him because we were seriously in debt. John turned the page over trying to hide it from me. He was too late. I had seen it. It was no good, I had to do something more. I had to take total responsibility for the family. I would start with the mortgage.

The next morning I rushed to the car, hurriedly put the toddlers into their car seats, put the double buggy into the boot and drove to town. I finally found a parking space in town, opened my car door, went to the boot, hauled out the double buggy and opened it up.

'Out you come,' I said, as I lifted the girls out one by one. 'Penny, stand next to the buggy while I get Emma.' Penny pulled at the handle of the double buggy while I extricated Emma from her seat. I locked all the car doors and put my hands on the handles of the double buggy.

'Right, climb in girls,' I said and the toddlers climbed into the chairs. Emma kicked her legs. 'Keep your feet still Emma or you will hurt yourself.' I pushed the buggy quickly before the girls thought up any more distractions.

There was a long queue at the bank. Penny was impatient.

'Out, I want out,' she said pushing herself up in the chair.

'No! You stay there!' I snapped.

Penny's mouth opened and a loud piercing wail filled the room. Emma joined in. The sound was deafening.

'Would you like to come forward?' One of the assistants, a slim blond, shouted above the noise. I pushed the buggy forward, the queue leaning back as the screams of the toddlers assailed their ears.

'How can I help you?' the assistant shouted above the noise, forcing a smile, her bright lipstick contrasting with her light blond hair.

I explained who I was. 'I need to be responsible for our mortgage,' I said.

The blond beckoned us into the office. She left the room for a moment and returned with a file. She smiled.

'No, I see that is not possible. Your husband has to be responsible.'

'But *I* have to pay the mortgage now!' I replied.

'Why?'

'Because my husband is ill.'

Penny stood up in her seat. I gently pushed her down, snatching one of the pamphlets from the desk and giving it to her. Emma snatched it and before Penny could cry I thrust another pamphlet into her little hands. The toddlers admired their prizes and crumpled them, making the shiny paper flash in the harsh light of the room.

The blond sat at the desk perusing the paperwork.

'No, I am sorry, you simply cannot be responsible for the mortgage.'

'Why not, for goodness sake? We *are* married.'

'I'm afraid the only way you can become responsible for the mortgage is if you leave you husband.'

'If I *leave* him? But the very reason I want to do it is because I want to help him, not leave him! If he weren't ill I wouldn't be here. What kind of nonsense is that?'

'I am sorry,' the blond flashed an insincere smile, 'that's that way it is.'

'Well I've never heard anything like it before!' I snorted. The girls jolted back into their seats as I turned the buggy round hurriedly and swept out of the room.

That was the first of many such brushes with bureaucracy. Harriet Bendall had already been doing her bit by feigning to assist but actually achieving nothing at all. Her self-important platitudes were incredible. Clearly I was not going to get any help at a time when we all needed it. I thought of my father in Australia. He was not getting any younger.

I changed up a gear and the car sped forward. There was quite a lot of traffic on the road but it was not the rush hour quite yet. The girls were safely with the child minder and I was in good time for school. The hum of the engine and the heat soothed my anxious spirit. The windscreen wipers moved hypnotically to and fro, to and fro. My eyes were tired. My head drooped. I jolted suddenly awake. This was not happening. I was not going to sleep. My eyes glazed and for a second I did not see the road. A horn blasted from behind me. I jolted again, shook my head, leaned forward and willed myself to concentrate on the splashes of rain on the road. It was getting too dangerous.

I gripped the wheel firmly. Only one more week to go before the holidays would come and I would finally be able to sleep. I struggled through the week and eventually the day of the great lie-in came. I did not have to leap out of bed, scramble to get the children washed, fed and dressed. I could lie in the bed for hours. I opened my eyes a little, stretched and closed my eyes again.

Suddenly from the room opposite, Penny screamed. Emma had gone into Penny's room to create havoc.

'John!' I said giving my husband a gentle push.

'They'll be all right,' he snapped. He had his back to me so his voice was subdued 'Leave them!'

I struggled out of bed and in a daze stumbled towards Penny's room.

'Girls, stop it!' I shouted.

Emma scuttled out of Penny's room and back into her own.

'Stay there until it's time to get up!' I growled as I leaned against the wall on the landing between the two rooms, slid down and stayed in that position, half-sitting and half-lying. This can't go on, I thought.

'We need to go away for a holiday. All of us.' I was pushing the sheets into the washing machine, Penny and Emma were squabbling near the front door and John was standing in the kitchen holding the kettle. He filled the kettle with water from the cold-water tap.

'We always went to Butlin's when I was a child. The children would love it.' He put the kettle down on the kitchen top, plugged it in and switched it on. It gave a soft hissing sound that was almost covered up with the squeals from the girls as they fought over a toy snake.

'Wherever you want, John,' I sighed, 'Anywhere will do as long as I get a break.'

Chapter 25

The day of our Butlin's holiday finally arrived.

'It's almost not worth going,' I sighed as I folded all the clothes and pushed them into one of the four cases. 'There is so much preparation to do.'

John stood awkwardly, watching me.

'But once we are there the girls will be entertained. You will love it, you'll see.' Penny bumped into her dad as she tried to escape the clutches of her little sister.

'Dad!' Penny said and ran out of the room to chase Emma who ran into the sitting room and slammed the door shut.

'Let me in! Let me in!' Penny banged on the door.

'Yes, maybe we will be able to enjoy it,' I said, more in hope than conviction. 'All ready?' I got into the driving seat. 'Got everything you want? Now is the time to remember anything you have forgotten.'

I looked at John. He looked straight ahead. His scowling face reminded me how resentful he was that he had lost his driving licence.

Penny kicked the back of my seat.

'Stop kicking, Penny,' I barked. 'Right, we're going. Butlin's Clacton here we come.'

'Look at all those houses,' I shouted so that the girls could hear me in the back of the car. 'How many have black roofs?'

Penny said, 'I see one!'

Emma shouted, 'I see one!'

'Where?' Penny asked scathingly. 'You can't see any houses now, only trees.'

I could see Emma in the rear vision mirror, sulking and sucking her thumb.

'I feel sick,' John said. I checked the road and stole a glance at John. He was decidedly pale.

'We can't stop here!' I passed a little white mini. There was nowhere to stop. 'Open the window.'

John wound down the window and leaned out of the car and vomited.

'What's Daddy doing?' Penny asked.

'He'll be all right in a minute,' I said. 'Not long now. We'll stop for lunch soon. Hold on, John, I can see a restaurant ahead.'

I swept the car into the car park of the Little Chef, leaned across John to the glove compartment of the car, pulled out some tissues and thrust them onto his chest. 'Here, take these to clean yourself up.'

'I don't want any lunch,' John muttered.
I looked at his white face and clenched knuckles.

'No,' I said, 'you don't look too good but there's no reason why we shouldn't have lunch. Why don't you lie down outside and have a bit of a rest?'

John slowly unbuckled his seat belt, opened his car door, staggered to a patch of sunlit grass and lay down.

I swiftly unbuckled my seatbelt, flung open my door and leaped out.

'Come on, children, we'll go and have lunch.'

I looked over to John. He looked comfortable lying still on the grass. The sun was shining strongly.

'I'll just put a cloth over your dad's head so that he doesn't get sunstroke and then we'll go girls,' I said.

'Isn't Daddy coming too?' Penny took hold of my hand; Emma grasped the other hand, pulling back as she took one last look at her dad.

Lunch was a success. The girls were so engrossed in their huge sundaes that we had all forgotten about John for a moment.

The door to the restaurant flung open. A large middle-aged woman shouted.

'There's someone outside having a fit!'

'Oh, my goodness, John!' I jumped to my feet. 'Wait here girls. I'll come back in a minute.'

The rest of the afternoon was a jumbled kaleidoscope of medics, ambulance, whining children, hospital and, finally, a late arrival at Butlin's.

'You're too late.' A fat worker swept the floor lazily. 'All's finished for the night.'

'But —' I stood, open-mouthed.

'You could try and ask the kitchens to call one of the managers if you like.' He kept on sweeping.

With the two girls clutching my hands, I asked, 'Where are the kitchens?'

The worker gestured lazily, pointing to the right, 'Over there.'

He turned his back and kept sweeping. The children and I arrived at what might have been the kitchens, but the kitchen doors were firmly closed.

'Can someone help us, please?' I asked to the darkened room. I could see some staff through glass doors at the side. They either did not hear me or decided I was indeed too late to be booked in.

'All right, girls, don't be too alarmed. I'm going to have a wobbly.'

'A wobbly? What's that, Mum?' Penny asked.

I took in a deep breath. 'Just watch,' I said, and screamed at the top of my voice: 'Will someone bloody well come and help us? My husband has been rushed to hospital and I have two tired children to see to.'

Figures behind the glass door froze. Two of them advanced quickly towards me.

'Is something the matter?' one of them asked. I bit my lip and put my arms around my crying children.

John slowly pulled himself out of his depression, and had been free of fits long enough to get his driving licence back. He even got a new job. Our family resumed its normal routine, John and I resumed our banter and John's jokes and his quirky sayings began to integrate themselves into the conversation. I could deal with his bad moods that seemed to come and go at a whim.

One sunny afternoon, I was washing up. The girls had gone to play with Babs' children in the next village and I was thinking how it was so good to be back to normal. The worst was over. John was taking his medication and seeing the doctor regularly. Although I was always tired and in need of a break, I felt I was managing. John looked after our finances, although I had long ceased trying to get any housekeeping from him. My salary was just covering the mortgage and our living expenses. The bank manager was keeping an eye on John's spending. His boss was looking after him at work for the moment. If the worst happened I would have to be the sole breadwinner. Everything will be all right.

The door rattled. The Saturday afternoon post had come. John was out working, or seeing his mother, I didn't mind which. At least he was happy, unless she threw one of her tantrums. He never told me when she did.

I picked up the post and scanned the envelopes. One of them was from the bank. We weren't expecting a statement. I was curious. It was addressed to both of us, so it must be about our joint account.

When I opened the letter I froze. 'This is our third and final letter...' *Third* letter? I did not remember receiving a first or a second letter. John had been hiding the mail again. Trembling I held it in my hands and paced the sitting room floor. This was terrible. When was John coming home? We must sort it out immediately.

I waited impatiently. Finally, the front door opened. John came into the hall, put his jacket on the coat hanger, hung it on the second peg from the left, brushed the lapels and paused in the sunlight streaming through the front door.

At the sound of his entrance, I shoved the letter quickly into my pocket, rushed into the kitchen and switched on the kettle. As I came out I straightened my cardigan and forced a smile on my pale face.

'Welcome home, dear,' I said as I stepped into my husband's sight. The room filled with sunlight. The afternoon was always the best time to enjoy a moment of relaxation in our sitting room. 'Would you like a cup of tea?' I asked.

'Yes, thanks, but make it properly will you?' he growled. He sat down in his armchair and picked up the newspaper on the table next to him. 'None of your usual bushwhacker stuff.' He began to read the front page.

'All right, don't worry; I'll warm the pot first.' I stepped lightly back into the kitchen, finally brought the tea tray out into the sitting room and placed it on the table.

'Where are the children?' he asked.

'They've gone to Babs for the afternoon.' I poured milk into the two china cups.

John turned over the first page of the newspaper and glanced at the headlines inside. 'More murder and mayhem in the cities, I see.'

'How has work been this week?' I failed to prevent the slight tremor in my voice.

'Fine, absolutely fine,' he said absently, folding the newspaper and returning it to the table. 'I'll get a tremendous bonus this year.' He took off the teapot cover and put it down on the table. He lifted up the teapot lid and looked inside. 'Not brewed yet. We'll leave it for a few moments.' He replaced the lid.

'I could give it a stir with a spoon,' I suggested.

'And stir up trouble? No, we'll wait.' John's voice hardened. A large truck rattled its way along the road outside the house.

I sat back in my chair biting my lip. I picked up my cup and put it down again. I spoke slowly and quietly.

'We received a letter today,' I said tentatively.

'We're always getting letters.' His eyes focused on the newspaper.

'This one is important.' I raised the tone of my voice one notch.

'They're all important to you,' he muttered. He crushed the newspaper onto his knee and looked at me directly. 'Come on, woman, what is it? Get it over and done with.'

'It's from the bank.'

'So?'

'It's about our joint account.'

John sighed. 'You know I have always said that you can take as much money as you like from our joint account.' He checked the teapot again. 'Shall I be mum? It's ready now.' He poured some tea into the two cups.

'We owe over a thousand pounds,' I blurted.

'So? I'll soon make it up with the bonus. Don't you worry your pretty head about it.'

'But I do!' I cried.

'Well, you shouldn't and that's the end of the matter.' He picked up his cup, sat back in his chair and took a sip.

I picked up my cup and put it down again.

'But there's more.'

John turned to face me. 'Oh, for goodness sake! What else could there be?'

'I received a visit today from your colleague, Ralph Johnson.'

'So, what could *he* want?' John placed his cup carefully in his saucer.

'He said that you are having difficulties at work.'

'Nonsense. I'm doing fine.' John's cup rattled.

'That's not what I heard from Ralph.' I gripped the edge of my chair.

'What would *he* know, anyway?' John slammed his cup and saucer down on the table. Tea splashed into the saucer and onto his knee. 'Now look what you've made me do!' He took out a white handkerchief from his trouser pocket and wiped the tea stain hurriedly.

'Ralph is your boss, isn't he? He said you aren't seeing enough customers.'

'I *am* seeing enough customers. I go out every day and come back late, don't I?' He pushed the handkerchief back into his pocket.

I shifted forward and glared at my husband. 'What about all the times you have been visiting your mother? Shouldn't you have been seeing customers then?'

John met my stare. 'You've always been jealous of her. I've told you and I'll tell you again, I'll see my mother as often as I like.'

I opened the palms of my hands and held them towards John, hoping the gesture would calm my petulant spouse.

'Look, John, of course you must see your mother. I'm not jealous of her, but you have your responsibilities here. If you're in trouble, all you have to do is confide in me. Perhaps I can help?'

John clenched his fists. 'I tell you there is nothing wrong. Now butt out.'

I held my ground. 'Wasn't there some trouble at the exhibition?'

'What would you know about it?' he snarled.

'Well, tell me. You shouldn't bottle it up like you do. What happened?' I stared at him. His eyes flickered. He was like a wounded animal, cornered.

'Some of these customers don't know what they are talking about,' he sneered. 'I told one of them where to get off, that's all.' He shifted his position uneasily in the chair. He would not meet my eyes. I sat back a little. Softening my voice, I asked:

'There's more, isn't there? About London?'

'London?' he paused as if weighing up carefully what he was going to say next. He sighed. 'Oh, they want us to move to Dagenham, that's all,' he mumbled.

I tried to keep the panic out of my voice. 'Why didn't you say anything about it before? Do you want to move to Dagenham?'

John paused. Finally he murmured, 'I'm not sure.'

'Right,' I said, grabbing the tea things and shoving them roughly onto the tray.

'That's enough.' I stood up, bent down quickly and strained to lift the tray. 'There's no way I'm going to take the children out of this area. We live in the countryside where the girls are happy and can play safely outside. We are not going to live in a small flat in the smog of London. It's no life for the children.' I rattled the teacups as I stumbled to the kitchen and dumped them on the draining board. 'You can go to London if you like, but you go on your own! Besides,' I shouted, making sure my voice reached from the kitchen to the sitting room, 'it's just their way of trying to get rid of you. Don't you realize that?'

John leaped to his feet and stormed out of the room. He grabbed his coat, opened the front door and slammed it behind him.

'That's right.' My lips curled with venom. 'Run to Mother!'

Chapter 26

We settled back into an uneasy routine. I felt I was living on a tightrope, juggling to keep us all dressed and fed and trying to keep down a full-time job.

'I've decided to join a different firm.' John stood in the kitchen. I was dishing up the dinner. I said nothing.

'I'm going to work for Thomas's.'

'Thomas's?' I asked, straining the vegetables and dishing then out on the plate.

'Yes. I'm on commission.'

'Not a salary?'

'No, they offer commission only these days'

I turned to look at him. His eyes were wide with apprehension.

'Well, as long as you're happy. Here, can you take these through to the dining room.' I handed him the girls' plates and walked to the playroom.

'Come on, girls. Dinner time.'

'Daddy is going to work for a new firm,' I said to the girls, trying to sound cheerful.

'I don't like peas,' Emma said.

'Well, just have a few,' I said, putting a fork full of carrots into my mouth and chewing swiftly.

John leaned over to Emma and snarled. 'Eat!'

Emma curled her lip and stared at her plate.

'Come on,' John persisted. 'Now!' He took the spoon out of her hand, filled it with peas and handed it to her. 'Take this and eat it!'

Tears flowed down her cheeks as Emma slowly grasped the spoon in her little fingers and put it to her lips. In choking gulps she ate a few of the peas from her spoon, staring at her father as she did so.

'You too, Penny!' he growled.

Penny quickly picked up her spoon, put a few peas on it and ate them, staring at her plate the whole time.

'You'll be doing a bit of travelling, I guess,' I said, forcing myself to keep the tone light.

'Probably,' John said. Then he pushed his plate forward. 'I'm not hungry. I'm going upstairs to do a bit of work' He stood up. The girls' eyes fixed on him as he left the dining room.

'It's all right, girls,' I sighed. 'Finish what you can, and then you can go to the playroom.'

The following Monday, John came in late from his new job.

'Mother is going on a cruise this Christmas,' he said as he came in the door.

'Welcome home, dear.' I gave him a peck on his lips, wondering how much real work he had done that day - for he had clearly spent the afternoon with his mother again. 'That will be nice for her,' I tried to disguise the sarcasm.

'I'll give her a lift to the dock.'

'How was work?'

'Oh, fine. I've got to keep the equipment in the car. I'll move it out into my office so that I can fit mother's case in the boot.'

John sat down on his chair in the sitting room. He looked pale. I wished he didn't feel obliged to accommodate his mother so readily. He had enough to worry about here at home.

'I'll check on the girls and get the tea,' I said. I went to the playroom. The girls were both concentrating on different toys at different ends of the playroom. I smiled. It was lovely to see their little fingers so busy, so happy. I went back into the kitchen.

Suddenly, there was a loud thump in the sitting room. I rushed into the room. John was lying on his side on the floor, his body convulsing. I knelt down to him and waited until the convulsing had stopped. He was finally still, breathing heavily.

I rushed to the phone and dialled. 'John has had another fit. Please come,' I said quickly.

A few minutes later the doorbell rang. The doctor stepped into the house quickly and went to John. John's eyes were open.

'John, are you all right?'

'Yesh.' John sounded drugged as he replied. The doctor helped John as he got to his feet. John walked unsteadily but purposefully towards the toilet. He closed the door behind him.

'Don't lock the door!' the doctor and I said in chorus. The door clicked. The doctor and I looked at each other. We waited. The toilet flushed and the door clicked open. John walked to his chair in the sitting room and sat down.

'It's all right,' the doctor patted my hand. 'I'll stay until he is properly out of the fit.'

'Mum?' Penny called from the hallway. 'I'm coming,' I called back and swiftly went to Penny and encouraged her back to the playroom.

The following morning John looked exhausted but he had dressed in his suit. He walked to the front door, put his briefcase down and turned to me for his usual peck on his cheek.

'Should you be going to work today?'

'Of course, why not?'

'Well, after the fit you had yesterday.'

'What of it? I don't remember anything about it.'

'What about the change of medication? Shouldn't you make sure that is OK? What if you have a fit while you are driving?'

'That's my lookout.'

'Yeah, but what about the other people on the road?'

'Look, it's all right. I'm popping into the doctor's first and then off to work?'

He picked up his briefcase, grabbed his jacket and swept out of the door.

A few hours later he came back. His mouth drooped. Something was amiss.

'Okay, spit it out. What's happened?' I tried to sound casual.

'The doc,' he grumbled.

'Yes? It's great that he is keeping an eye on you, isn't it?'

'He is writing to the Vehicle Licensing Authority. He's going to get my driving licence revoked.'

I stopped folding the clean clothes from the laundry basket and turned to him.

'Oh, I *am* sorry.'

'It won't be for long. I can get it back if I have been fit free for a year.'

'It's lucky that I drive, isn't it?'

He did not reply. He turned and went slowly upstairs to his office.

Two years passed and both girls were on the verge of going to school. John had failed to remain fit-free long enough to get his licence back. He had busied himself in the neighbourhood, but there was always an underlying feeling that he had let us down. He felt he should to be the breadwinner no matter what, and he resented my full-time job and the fact that I could drive. I could hardly wait for the day the girls would be going to school, so they could experience a different life.

'Now,' I said to John, who was keen to play Dad, taking them to school. 'You must be on time and stay with them until the teacher comes out.'

'Of course,' he said with a twinkle in his eye. 'I'll be there with all those good-looking mums.'

I glanced at him. 'And when you collect them after school on Fridays, would you like to take them to the shop to buy some sweets as a treat for them?'

'That's a good idea. I'll get something for us too,' he grinned.

'And about the lawns.' I was getting everything packed in now he was in a good mood. 'You are supposed to mow the lawns every Saturday. You said you would. They haven't been cut for two weeks. You will do the lawns this Saturday?'

'Anything for a quiet life,' he groaned. The lawns remained untouched that Saturday.

'It is the least you can do,' I shouted. 'I've been out to work every day this week, I get the meals, get the girls ready for school; I do nearly everything and you can't even mow the lawns. It's not fair!'

John stared at me, impervious to my anger. He'd heard it all before.

'Why do I put up with it?' I murmured under my breath.

Chapter 27

The brown envelope looked innocuous enough. At least it's not a bill, I thought, as I read the contents. But it was worse. The busybody Harriet Bendall was calling a meeting about John at the Institute of Health. I was invited to attend.

After a great deal of organization, John, the children and cover at work were sorted and I drove to the Institute.

'Could you please tell me where room Eight is?' I asked the petite receptionist. 'I have an appointment with Miss Bendall.'

'It's down the corridor and first on the right,' she said, pointing in that direction.

I knocked on the door.

'Come in,' a confident voice called.

I stepped into the room. It was full of people. Ten pairs of eyes stared at me.

'Mrs Wilks, about John Wilks?' I asked tentatively. I could not believe that so many people needed to be there to talk about John.

'Ah, yes,' Harriet said. Her slim suit and the haughty position of her head at the centre of the group left no doubt that she was going to run the meeting. 'Yes, he is on the agenda.' She said crisply. 'Please sit down.' She waved her hand towards an empty chair in the corner of the room.

I sat down.

The woman sitting immediately in front of me turned round. 'Do pull up your chair and join us,' she said to me, almost in a whisper.

I picked up the chair and squeezed it between her and a thin middle-aged man.

'   'Well then, Mrs Wilks,' Harriet said, 'as you know, I am Harriet Bendall and I am chair of this meeting.' She turned to her group. 'Let's look at agenda item Nine. John Wilks was added to our list four weeks ago. Is there anything to report?'

An assistant in beige, wearing the largest spectacles I had ever seen, said, 'Dr Young is pleased with his progress. He seems settled at home and there have been no incidents lately.'

After a brief non-report from the other individuals, Miss Bendall turned her attention to me.

'Is there anything you have to say, Mrs Wilks?'

I cleared my throat. 'I am worried that I cannot cope with John as well as I should. I feel he could do something dangerous at any moment.'

'Well, I am sure we are doing everything we can. You do realize that a patient has to be seriously ill before we could consider doing any more than we are already, don't you?'

I blushed but forced myself to look straight into her steely eyes. She did not blink.

'Well, I think that covers John Wilks,' she snapped, firmly closing the file in front of her. 'Thank you for attending, Mrs Wilks. We won't keep you any longer. Now about Mrs Abbott ...'

I stumbled out of the room muttering, 'That was a waste of time!' and rushed to my car.

I had a restless night. John came home late and we were barely civil to each other when we spoke.

The following evening there was a knock on the door.

'Good evening.' A cheery middle-aged woman held out her card. 'I'm Mrs Abbott, the social worker. I believe you have had a meeting with the famous Harriet Bendall. I've come to see if I can help.'

I swept open the door quickly, 'Please come in.' Wasn't Abbott the name of the person Miss Bendall mentioned at the end of our meeting? I was curious. I opened the sitting room door and indicated the only seat that was free from the children's toys.

'Sorry about the mess,' I murmured as Mrs Abbott carefully stepped over the Lego bricks, a small train set in pieces, dolls, cushions and other paraphernalia that surrounded the youngsters. She sat down.

'Is John here?' she asked.

I held Emma's arm, as she was about to hit her sister in an argument over the train. 'No, he's gone next door.'

Mrs Abbott shifted back into her chair. 'That's probably for the best. We can talk freely.'

Satisfied that the girls were now well apart and interested in different piles of toys, I sat down.

'Can we have some help?'

'You certainly look as though you need some help. Unfortunately, Harriet Bendall, the woman in charge of your case, says it isn't possible. Funding, you know.'

I grimaced. But of course, what else could I expect?

Mrs Abbott continued, 'I'm leaving the Social Services next week, so I can tell you the only way you can get help.'

I sat forward. 'And what is that?'

Mrs Abbott glanced at the girls who were both concentrating hard on other things. They were not listening. She lowered her voice. 'The only way you can get the authorities to help is to pack up your things and take the children and yourself to stay with a friend. Then ring up the authorities and say that your husband is alone in the house, that he is a danger to himself and others and he's their responsibility.'

I paled. 'No! We can't do that, surely!'

Mrs Abbott shrugged. 'I'm afraid that's the only way I know of that works. That's why I'm leaving Social Services. So many people like yourself are in desperate need of help and are just not getting it.'

I stood up. 'Well, I suppose I should thank you for being so candid. Would you like a cup of tea or something?'

Mrs Abbott stood. 'No, thank you. I must get on. I hope you get some help.' She walked to the front door. I opened it for her and waved to her as she walked to her car.

Penny squawked with frustration. I rushed back to the sitting room. One of the lids Penny was holding would not fit on one of the tins. 'No, it belongs to another tin,' I said as I grabbed the other tin and gave the tin and the lid to Penny. Penny's little fingers finally put the lid on the tin. She grinned. Emma picked up another tin and separate lid, tried to copy her sister, soon gave up and tossed them aside. She picked up a large ball and shook it, putting it to her ear so that she could hear the jingles.

I sat down heavily on my chair. What was I to do? Friends had said that the three of us could stay at their house at the last minute if John became too difficult. But could I leave my husband like that? I went upstairs to find sleeping bags and a change of clothes for the three of us. I felt guilty. It seemed wrong to plan to escape from my husband. We married for better or for worse. Then I remembered the last time I had seen his face contorted with anger over some trivial matter. I quickly dashed downstairs and put the bags in the boot of the car, ready. My fingers trembled as I put the last one into the boot and shut it. I bit my lip; my heart was heavy with guilt. It was like a betrayal, a resignation, the beginning of the end. I went inside and sat with the children. Tears welled up in my eyes.

The canons in Tchaikovsky's 1812 overture brought me back to the present. John, my bed-ridden husband lay inert. The overture came to a halt; a soothing voice announced the next piece of classical music on the radio.

'Well, I don't know,' I said to the figure slumped in front of me, 'you were always one to choose your moments, weren't you?'

John made a muted noise. I knew it was not really a reply; it was just something for him to do. He kept making the noises while I continued to talk.

'I finally realized that whenever we did anything different, you were likely to have one of your fits. You seemed to have one during every holiday we had, didn't you?'

He yawned.

'There was a time when I nearly left you.' He did not respond. 'Fortunately I'm not sure that you fully understand what I'm saying at the moment, so I guess it won't matter if I tell you now.'

'It was the time just after I managed to get work and you had lost one of your jobs. I didn't realize it then, but your illness had started. I couldn't get through to you.'

I paused and looked out of the window at the clear blue sky. 'You know, the sky was the same colour that day.'

The summer holidays came. We were having a very late breakfast in the dining room. John had finished his single piece of toast and had left the table.

'I'm going to the post office,' he called as he went out the front door. At least he's going somewhere, I thought to myself.

I spoke to the girls. 'I have something important to say.' The girls looked enquiringly, their young faces assuming a wise and knowledgeable look for the ages of 5 and 6.

'I am going to say some terrible things, but you must not be upset. To make the authorities help your dad, I'm going to say that I'm going to Australia. I'm going to have to sound as if I really mean it, but I promise you I will never leave you. You will be all right.' Tears welled up in their eyes.

'All right, Mum,' they murmured, their heads bowed.

'You can go and play now.' The girls jumped down from their chairs swiftly and raced into the playroom nearby.

I sighed and started clearing up the breakfast things. There was a knock on the door.

A slim lady in a suit frowned at me.

'Mrs Wilks?' she asked.

I looked up and down the well-groomed figure. Oh no! Not the horrid Harriet Bendall. She certainly wasn't caring for young children at the moment. I put my hand to my hair, wondering when I last had a chance to brush it.

'Yes, that's me.' I looked at her defiantly. 'What do you want?'

'Remember, I'm Harriet Bendall, in charge of your husband's case?' She offered a limp hand to shake. 'I have been instructed by the committee to pay you a home visit. Well, are you going to invite me in?' She stepped forward. I touched the handle briefly and pulled the door back slowly.

Miss Bendall stepped quickly across the threshold, lifted her dainty feet over the coats that had fallen down in her path, marched into the sitting room, cleared the newspaper off one of the chairs and sat down.

I sat opposite her and said abruptly, 'We need help. John's behaviour is getting more aggressive and erratic. What are you going to do to help us?'

Harriet's eyes glassed over. 'It's impossible. You are coping perfectly so —'

I interrupted, 'If you are not going to help, I may as well go to Australia. My father needs me just as much.' My voice was increasing in pitch until it had reached a penetrating shrillness that took me by surprise.

Harriet pursed her lips. 'Well, if you really can't cope, we will take the children into care.'

I sat bolt upright. 'Into care?' I was stunned. 'How *could* you?'

She stood up and said, as she walked to the door, 'I have many other people to see, I'm sorry but I must go.'

Still reeling from the new threat I went to the door and opened it. I said nothing as Harriet swept through the doorway and walked smartly to her car. I shut the door slowly and went to sit down again. So, now they will take the children into care! This is *not* going to happen. I went upstairs to my computer and started making lists of exactly who was looking after the children and when. In order to do my job, there were times when someone needed to look after the children. If the children were in bed at night, John was all right, but left on his own with the tension their bickering created ... I decided that I would try not to leave him alone with them for too long.

Some keys rattled in the front door and it opened. John had returned from the post office. As I was finishing the first list of where we were going and who was looking after the children every minute of the day when I was at work, there was a loud clatter and a scream coming from downstairs. Now what?

'John?' I called. But John did not reply. I ran downstairs and saw him seated at the desk in the sitting room, writing. I rushed passed him, through the kitchen and dining room to the playroom. One of the chairs near the entrance had been knocked over. Emma was gripping her leg and crying. I looked at the leg. It seemed all right, there were no cuts and she could move it.

I snarled, 'Can't you play for a few moments without interrupting me?' I bit my lip. I had not meant to be so abrasive. Emma cried even more. Penny looked up from her pile of Lego, surprised by the tone of her mother's voice.

I quickly leant down to Emma, rubbed the leg then hugged her saying with a much kinder tone, 'There there, better soon.' I clutched Emma tighter, turned my head to the side and let the tears fall for a brief moment before quickly releasing her, brushing the tears from my cheeks and rushing out of the playroom before the children noticed my tears.

I walked through the dining room and into the kitchen where I could hear the girls clearly, folded my arms and leant against the wall. Things could not go on like this much longer. It felt as though I were on my own, isolated, with three troublesome individuals who constantly needed the attention I could not provide. I sniffed and reached for a kitchen towel. I yearned for someone to hold me, to comfort me and say that everything would be all right. That night I dreamed of Dennis Parker. His arms were round me. I argued with him but he ignored my pleas and pulled me to him ... I awoke with a jolt. The bathroom door slammed. John was going to the toilet.

I turned my bedside light on. No, Dennis was not the answer. He already had a wife. I suddenly wanted my dad. Maybe I *would* take the children to Australia to be with Dad after all? Yes, I would leave John and take the children with me. The authorities would then *have* to help him, the children would be able to get to know their granddad and I could resume my teaching career there. I snuggled back under the bedclothes and started planning.

Chapter 28

The next night, late, after the children were in bed and John was asleep I went downstairs and picked up the phone.

'Yes?'

'Dad? It's me,' I croaked.

'Hello, Sally? How are you?'

'Not good,' I gulped.

'Oh, Sally,' my father's tone was low, sympathetic. My tears flowed freely.

'I'm leaving him,' I blubbered. 'Can the girls and I come and stay with you?'

My father said immediately, 'Of course you can. I can put in an extra bathroom ...'

'Oh, Dad, that's all I wanted to hear. I'll ring you again after I've got things organized.'

I put the phone down, dragged my exhausted body through the motions of getting ready for bed, climbed under the sheets and fell sound asleep.

When I awoke the next morning, I could hear a blackbird singing its heart out in the bright morning light. What had I done? John was quiet. The girls were also sound asleep. Were things as bad as I had imagined? The tell-tale thud of little feet on the bedroom floor interrupted my thoughts. I had to get up and see to the children, sort out my husband before getting ready for work, get the dinner organized for when they got home...

'Don't!' Penny screamed from her room. 'Go away!'

I sighed and forced myself out of bed.

'Stop it, girls,' I called. They knew their mum was too exhausted to chase up her words with action.

'Get off!' Emma snarled. I could hear more thumping from Penny's room. There were no serious screams yet.

'Anyway, I've got the bathroom first!' Penny shouted, scuttling into the bathroom and slamming the door loudly. I lay back for a moment. I looked at the bedroom clock. Just one more minute I murmured, closing my eyes.

'I'm going to leave John,' I said, looking down into my coffee as though it were absorbing the enormity of what I said. 'I'm not getting any help with him.'

'Oh, I am sorry.' Babs put her hand gently on top of mine. Babs, stalwart of friends, had called in that Sunday to see how we all were. We were sitting in the dining room within easy earshot of the children who were crashing about noisily but happily in the playroom.

I stirred my coffee for the third time. 'He needs supervision. He's getting worse.'

Babs took a sip of her coffee and put her mug down.

'Why, what's happening?'

'He — '

John stumbled into the dining room. 'You two ladies taking time off again?'

I stood up. 'Do you want a coffee? Do you want to join us?'

John stepped forward. 'No. Babs, you must know cars are breaking the speed limit down Common Road.

The council ought to do something about it. All those overpaid council workers sitting on their backsides doing nothing. It's about time something was done.'

Babs, somewhat bemused said, 'Er, yes, John.' He turned and left the room.

'You see,' I said. 'He's always lecturing everyone about irrelevancies. But more worryingly, when I go out of an evening for a break, the children say he is angry all the time. He clips them around their ears — not enough to really hurt them — but he seems to be getting worse and worse.'

'Oh, dear. What does his doctor say?'

'I take him to the doctor when he does something particularly strange and the doctor says there is nothing wrong. If I go to Australia, at least my dad will be supportive.'

One of the children shrieked, 'It's mine! Give it to me!' There was a loud crash.

I leapt to my feet and rushed to the playroom. Penny was pushing Emma hard. Emma was fighting back still clutching a book.

I marched over to the girls, snatched the book and shouted, 'If you can't share this book, I will take it away. Now behave yourselves. Why don't you go outside into the garden?'

Penny poked her tongue out at her sister, opened the back door and went outside. Emma sat sulking in the chaos of the playroom. I returned to my cold coffee. Babs stared into her mug.

'But it would be a tremendous upheaval for you all if you go to Australia.'

'I know. I suppose at my age I ought to be able to cope with whatever problems come my way.'

Babs looked at me, waiting for me to put my thoughts together.

I continued, 'It would be unfair of me to inflict my problems on poor ol' Dad I guess. Maybe I'll stay.'

Babs leaned forward. 'Better the devil you know, eh? You know you can always call on me to babysit, or even John-sit if you need.'

I sighed. 'Oh, thank you, Babs. John-sit? That would be lovely. You are such a great friend.' Tears welled in my eyes.

'It's all right, don't you worry. Now why don't you go upstairs and have a rest while I supervise the girls and John for a little?'

I stood up. 'Oh thank you. I will. Wake me up if I'm asleep too long.'

I left the dining room. Babs picked up the two mugs and headed for the kitchen sink. As I walked past the sitting room I could see John at the desk. He was writing another of his long letters. At least someone else was getting the brunt of his 'verbal diarrhoea' as he called it.

'Stop kicking me!' Penny shouted. It was a sunny Saturday afternoon in May and the girls were playing in the garden. Penny shoved Emma into a rose bush.

'That hurt!' Penny shrieked, as she disentangled herself from the thorns. She poked her tongue out at her sister.

'I'll do what I like,' Emma said, giving Penny a shove, and they fell in a heap on the damp grass, a tangle of arms, legs and hair.

I ran to them. 'Really, girls, you must learn to be kinder to each other. Now come on!' Grabbing an arm of each girl, I separated them and glared at each one in turn. They faced each other, their faces like thunder.

'Right, there is nothing for it, you will go to Sunday school tomorrow and learn a little about what is right and wrong and how to treat each other!'

The next day, Sunday, John stood at the bedroom door.

'I rang Mother yesterday. We're going to visit her for afternoon tea,' he said in that authoritative tone that I had learnt not to ignore. 'Now that I've got my driving licence back, I'll drive us there.'

My heart started thumping. My mother-in-law. Why did even the sound of her name cause me such anxiety? It was not as if we fought or even had an argument. She was always so cold, so still.

'I suppose we haven't seen her for a few months,' I sighed. 'All right then,' I said, as I climbed slowly out of bed. I could have done with some extra sleep. I looked at the clock. It was an hour earlier than I needed to get up to get the girls ready for their compulsory Sunday school.

My stomach gripped and I could not prevent the feeling of nausea that threatened to overwhelm me. But I knew this nausea was not physical, it was a psychological dread of afternoon tea with my mother-in-law. Would she be the charming person I had seen when other people were with us? Or would this visit be one of those emotional outbursts when she believed the world and her family was conspiring to make her life horrible?

Sunday school, Sunday lunch and the huge pile of washing up were glimpses in my thoughts as I tried to calm the anxiety that increased by the hour. It was only for a few hours in the afternoon, I tried to reason with myself, but nothing would stop the heavy feelings that were overwhelming me.

We were eventually in the car. John, smiling, drove us out into the road and turned towards Peterborough. I sat grimly next to him, determined to do all that I could to make the visit as pleasant as I could, even if it killed me.

The road was smooth and so far the journey was without mishap. I glanced in the rear-view mirror. Well, at least the girls were behaving reasonably well now. Then they began to fidget.

'Why don't you play 'I Spy' girls?' I suggested.

'All right,' said Penny, 'I'll start. I spy something beginning with —"c",' she said. Emma said, 'Car.'

Penny shouted, 'No!'

Emma tried 'Clock.'

Penny said, scathingly, 'There's no clock. Where can you see a clock?'

Emma sulked. 'On Daddy's wrist.'

'That's not a clock, that's a watch,' Penny shouted, grinning broadly. 'Do you give in?'

Emma was silent.

Penny repeated menacingly, 'Do you give in?'

The sound of the car engine altered as John changed gear.

Emma kicked the chair in front of her. 'All right, then, I give in.' Penny beamed.

'It's chimney!' Emma scowled.

'But that's not "c", that's "ch"!' Penny smirked. 'But the first letter of "ch" is "c". Na-na-na-na-na,' she chanted.

I intervened. 'Why don't you play another game? Why don't you see how many red cars pass by?'

John, driving with renewed confidence now that he had regained his driving licence, eased the car through the traffic in central Peterborough. My stomach began to tighten. As we came nearer to Mother-in-law's road, nausea swept over me. I swallowed and willed myself not to give in to the feelings of helplessness that threatened to overwhelm me.

John turned the wheel and we drove into the tidy cul-de-sac.

The garden was meticulous as expected. Every time I had seen it, there had never been a blade of grass or even a flower out of place. It was as if everything had been marshalled into line.

'We're here!' John said excitedly. He unbuckled his seatbelt and leaped out of the car.

I reluctantly opened my door, climbed out and shut it behind me. I opened the door behind me and let Penny out of her seatbelt and then Emma.

'Best behaviour, girls.' They stood behind me fidgeting. John rang the doorbell. We waited and after a considerable delay, the door opened slowly.

'You're late.' Mother-in-law's smooth features appeared in the open doorway.

'Come on, Mother,' John chirruped, 'let us in.'

Mother-in-law stepped back and led the way into the white-carpeted sitting room. It was as if the room had never been used, as if it was prepared as part of a show house. I looked at the girl's shoes. They should have taken them off at the front door. I hurriedly took them off and put them with my own and a pair of shoes already sitting by the front door.

'Have you got any toys?' Penny asked.

'No,' their granny said. 'Now let me have a look at you.' She sat on one of the large armchairs and beckoned the girls to come and stand in front of her.

I called to John who was making the tea in the kitchen, 'I'll come and give you some help, shall I?' I left the room and found John carefully laying out the bone china cups. There were some sandwiches and cakes placed neatly on the side. The sandwiches were cut in symmetrical shapes, their crusts missing.

'I'll carry these in, shall I?' I said nervously. I needed to keep my hands busy.

Eventually we were seated at the table. I glared at Penny and Emma and they took their arms off the table.

'Sally has to go to a summer conference in July,' John said, his voice light and cheery. His mother made no comment.

'I'll need some help with the girls,' John continued. 'Could you have the girls to stay with you for a short while?'

His mother stirred her tea. 'It would be very inconvenient. I have a lot of commitments, you know.'

John persisted. 'Not even just one of the girls to stay over a weekend?'

She stared at him, 'No.'

I bit my lip. I had to stop myself from blurting out, 'See! I told you!'

'Can we go outside?' Penny said fidgeting in her chair.

'Me too,' Emma wriggled in her seat.

No one spoke.

'Yes,' I said suddenly, 'but mind Granny's plants and don't tread on the grass. Keep to the paths.'

The girls dashed back to the front door, picked up their shoes, ran to the back door of the house, put their shoes on and dashed outside. I could hear their chatter as they made up their own game of jumping on and off the stones on the paths.

The car was silent on the way home. The girls had fallen asleep and I did not dare say anything to upset John while he was driving. I snuggled into my seat. At least I didn't have to see my mother-in-law for another six months or so.

Chapter 29

The beeps on the radio announced the news. John liked to listen to the news. I was suddenly brought back into the present, into John's room in the care home. I looked at the prone figure before me. John's eyes were fixed, unblinking. What was happening? I waved my hand in front of his eyes. He did not blink. I sat in silence.

It was just like the first time I had witnessed a student in my class in Tasmania having a petit mal seizure. He had been in mid-sentence and had stopped suddenly.

'And? 'I had said, urging him to finish his sentence. Some students were yelling too loudly at the back of the classroom. I turned to face them.

'Quiet!' I demanded in the penetrating teacher's voice I had developed thanks to our scruffy dog, which had taught me exactly the right tone to use. 'Get on with your work!' The class noise level decreased. The individual having the seizure finished his sentence and the lesson resumed.

John still did not move in his bed. Was *he* having a petit mal seizure? If so, he didn't understand anything and couldn't communicate. But how would I know whether he had stopped communicating now, when it was a struggle to communicate all the time? He must have been reacting to me in some way when he was not having a fit. His eyes changed. They focused. He was out of the fit.

'Well, at least you are in a kind of hospital now,' I sighed. 'And you've been in enough of those in your time, haven't you?' I patted his hand then walked to the table, picked up the photo album and went back to his bedside.

'Still, we had some good times, didn't we?' I opened the album. 'Look here you are on your bike.' I looked at John. He stared unblinkingly. 'That was in the days when you biked to work and I drove the children to school in the car.'

John had more fits, he lost his driving licence again and the fits were now having their effect. He had changed. He was on strong medication and sat about the house, lethargic, and unmotivated. I had never known him to be as bad as this before.

'Are you sure you are giving him the right medication? I asked the doctor.

'Let me see,' he perused the sheet he was holding in his lily-white fingers. 'Mm.'

I fidgeted. John sat next to me, numb. Why didn't the doctor answer my question?

The doctor wrote on the sheet and turned to face John. 'I think I'll refer you to hospital, John. We need to assess you properly.'

He turned to face me. 'There will be a bed for him next Wednesday. Take him in for 10.30.'

I leaned forward, opened my mouth for the next question, but the doctor had stood up, and began shepherding us out of the room.

The following Wednesday I grabbed the girls' coats. 'Come on, put your coats on. It's cold outside and we will have a long walk to Daddy's ward.' I grabbed John's hospital bag, and called to John, 'Come on, John, it's time to go.' The house was silent.

'Girls, wait here,' I snapped at Penny and Emma as they stood at the front door. I dumped John's hospital bag at their feet. 'I'll be back soon.' I stomped upstairs to our room. John was seated on the end of the bed, his hands firmly under his thighs.

'I'm here,' he said.

'Now, come on.' I used my schoolmarm voice. 'The hospital is waiting for you. It's only for a few days. You'll be coming back home soon.' I picked up his bag and handed it to him. 'We've really got to go now.'
He looked at me and at the bag. The girls were squabbling in the hall. He picked up his coat and followed me slowly down the stairs.

'Stop it!' I shouted at the girls as I picked up his hospital bag, waded through the children and opened the front door. 'Now go and stand next to the back door of the car and I'll let you in'. Penny gave Emma an extra shove and they walked reluctantly towards the car. The sky was covered in ominously dark clouds. I settled the girls in the back seats of the car and opened the passenger door for John. I sat in the driver's seat, started the engine and eased the car out of the drive.

The next day I was finishing the washing up after breakfast, listening to the radio.

'The temperature has dropped below zero. The roads are very icy. The police have issued a warning not to drive unless absolutely necessary.'

The phone rang.

'Mrs Wilks?

'Yes?' I lifted my voice above the radio commentator. I should have turned it off before answering the phone.

'It's Doctor Painton here.'

'Yes?'

'We would like you to come in to the hospital to see us. Can you manage it later this morning, in about an hour?'

My fingers trembled. There must be something seriously wrong. 'I suppose so, if it's important.'

'I'll see you then, at about 11 a.m., on John's ward.'

My mouth was dry, my hands shook. I threw a towel over the rest of the dishes I was about to dry and called to the children. I hated winter. It always took so long to get the girls ready to go out. I grabbed our coats and shoved some biscuits and tissues into my pockets.

Sky and earth joined in a fog of icy air. The trees that I could see were picture perfect, frozen in time with the touch of Jack Frost, icy fingers reaching into the fog.

'Be careful,' I said to Penny and Emma, taking their hands as they stepped onto the icy pavement outside. 'Take tiny steps.'

'I'm cold,' Penny whined. I fiddled with the car lock, my fingers frozen through the woollen gloves. I finally opened the car door, leaned into the back of the car and unlocked the back door. I stepped out of the car again and swung the door back. I went round the back of the car and opened the other back door. Penny and Emma climbed into their seats and I put on and locked their seat belts. Emma moaned. The whining noise she made went right through me. I snapped.

'You can stop whining. I don't want to drive in this weather either but the doctor said we must come. You want to see you daddy, don't you?' The back seat of the car was silent.

I grabbed the scraper and demister spray from the glove box and went outside the car again. I sprayed the front windscreen liberally and scraped off the ice. I repeated the exercise with the back windscreen. I climbed into the car again.

'Right, we're off at last,' I said as I turned the key in the ignition. The car would not start. I muttered under my breath. My nose was cold from the freezing air; clouds of steam came out of my mouth as I breathed.

'I want to get out,' Penny whined. Oh how I longed for the heater. Gritting my teeth, I turned the key again and held it, pushing my foot on the accelerator. Finally the car coughed into action.

I eased forward slowly. It was very slippery under the wheels. Our road had not been treated with salt, so I gripped the wheel firmly as I peered through the fog. Most drivers had heeded the warnings of the police so I had the road to myself. I turned the wheel slightly; the car immediately went into a skid. I let it ride it out and cautiously turned the wheel again as I headed for the safer, treated main road.

The journey to the hospital was tortuous; my shoulders ached with tension as I leaned over the wheel staring hard into the fog. The dim outline of the large hospital finally came into view. I parked. Cold, hungry and out of sorts I gathered the girls together and we walked carefully on the icy pavements towards the entrance. The heat from inside the hospital was heaven when it greeted us.

'I'm hungry,' wailed Emma.

'We'll find Daddy's ward first, and I'll give you something to eat afterwards.' I dragged the unwilling children towards John's ward.

'Dr Painton said he wanted to see us?' I asked the nurse who was busy with paperwork at the desk in the centre of the ward.

'Dr Painton? I'll see if he's here.' She looked distractedly over her shoulder. 'Please take a seat over there.' She pointed to a waiting area almost filled with the huddled figures of defeated human beings. An old man with drooping white whiskers coughed into his gloved hand. I handed Penny and Emma a biscuit each.

'You sit there, Penny, and you over there, Emma.' I sat in a seat where I could see both girls. I was not in the mood to try to read a magazine.

'When can we see Daddy?' Penny called to me.

'After we have seen the doctor,' I called back. The other patients frowned at us. They wanted to brood in silence, they did not want to be troubled with our tiny little world.

A sprightly man wafted into the waiting room, looked around at the brooding faces and beamed.
'Why, it's Sally!' I stared at him. His beaming face reminded me of John. Of course, it was Matthew Wilks. We had met at Granny's so long ago.

'Uncle Matthew!' I smiled. 'Do come and sit next to me.' I ignored the glare of the fat woman occupying part of Matthew's chair.

'How is John?' he asked. 'I'd heard he wasn't well.'

'Yes, he's had fits and has lost his driving licence. It's a bit of a worry but we'll get through it.'

'You know I'd help if I could. It's such a pity he didn't get Jim's farm. He would have been *so* happy as a farmer. Eunice —'

'The doctor will see you now,' the nurse called crisply to me. 'Room Five.' I looked longingly at Matthew. I wanted to talk, but the nurse stood over me with folded arms.

'Come on, girls,' I called as I stood up. If the doctor was ready to see us so soon, there must be something seriously wrong. What could it be?

'Who was that man?' Penny asked loudly.

'Uncle Matthew,' I snapped.

The door marked '5' opened and a young man in a white coat smiled at us. I ushered the children towards the door.

'Do come in and sit down,' he forced a smile at the children, squeezed into his cramped office.

My heart thumped against my chest. I sat on the chair opposite him; the girls stood either side of me.

'Thank you for coming.' The doctor glanced at the file he had in front of him.

'I wanted to say how we are doing all we can to find out what is wrong with your husband.'

I sat still, stunned.

'Don't you know?'

'We are carrying out the usual tests. I just wanted to make sure you knew that we had his interests in mind.' He quickly snatched the pen from Emma as she fiddled with it.

I reddened. 'You mean, you dragged us through the ice when the police advised us not to travel, just to say that!' my voiced grew louder and louder. 'Didn't you think what it would be like for us? Have you no understanding of the situation? And you can't even tell me what is wrong with him?'

Before he could speak, I grabbed the girls by their hands and swept to the nurse's desk. There was no sign of Uncle Matthew.

'Where is my husband, please? I want to see him so that this dangerous journey has not been a complete waste of time!' The nurse bit her lip and walked towards the end of the ward. She pointed to the cubicle on her left. John's eyes sparkled when he saw us. The girls climbed up and sat on the bed to be with their daddy. I watched their muddy shoes mark the blanket. I did nothing to stop them. That was the last time I was going to completely trust the medical profession.

Five days passed, the weather improved and we were at the hospital to bring John home.

'Well, what did you find out?' I asked the doctor.

'The brain scan was borderline. There was nothing definite. You can take him home and he is to continue taking the tablets.'

'Thank you,' I smiled through gritted teeth, trying to look pleased with their efforts, but where were we to go from here?

Chapter 30

A month later, I struggled to the front door with my heavy school bag. I put the key into the lock and opened the door. The children, their squabbling voices filling the air, battled their way in front of me. I was too tired to argue. I was looking forward to a cup of tea and a sit down. Thank goodness John could still make a cup of tea.

There was no one in the house. Where was he? He couldn't be at his mother's because he was not allowed to drive. Maybe someone had given him a lift? I shrugged my shoulders, dropped my schoolbag onto the sitting room floor by the desk and picked up the mail from the floor. John usually dealt with the mail. Perhaps he was wandering round the village, creating mischief? Well, the village would have to take care of him for the moment; I needed my cup of tea. I glanced through the mail, there was nothing important. I put it on the desk and went to the kitchen. The girls had dumped their bags at the front door, gone into the kitchen, grabbed a drink and a biscuit and shot upstairs. I ignored the debris they had left in the kitchen, put the kettle on, checked the phone for messages and leant on the kitchen sink while I waited for the kettle to boil.

'I'm home!' John's cheerful voice called. His cheeks were flushed and his eyes glistened from the cold wind from his cycle ride. 'And I've got a job.' He grinned.

'You *have*? Wonderful!' I cried and gave him a hug. His clothes needed a good wash. I decided I would have to deal with that at the weekend.

'Where?'

'At the packaging factory in the next village.'

'A factory job?' I tried to disguise the disappointment in my voice. John, the smartly dressed, assured salesman with the posh voice was reduced to a factory worker. It would not suit him. They would make fun of his posh ways. He was heading for trouble.

'Isn't that a bit far to cycle?'

'Not for me, it isn't.

'When do you start?'

'Tomorrow morning. I'm on the early shift this week. I leave before six so you'll have to pack my lunch for me tonight.'

'I like that,' I teased. '*You'll* have to pack *my* lunch — can't *you* do it?'

'You don't have a dog and bark yourself. Besides, you do the shopping and know what to give me.'

He hugged me again. I smiled. My shoulders relaxed. John would no longer be a burden in the house. I would not spend my teaching hours worrying about what he was getting up to. He would be with other people and under supervision. It would be all right. I could easily prepare a packed lunch while I got the dinner ready in the evening.

The next morning he got up before the children and me. I stretched in bed, savouring a few moments when I had the bed to myself and five more minutes before I had to get the children up, dress and feed them and let the exhausting scenario continue.

That afternoon, when the girls and I came home after school, John was in his chair in the sitting room, unshaved, un-showered and still wearing his outdoor coat and woolly hat. I said nothing. He had a job and pride was restored now that he was contributing to the household expenses (or at least paying off some of his debt). One thing at a time, I told myself. Besides, the girls needed my attention.

In the fourth week, John's shift had changed back to the early time so he was home when we got back from school every night.

'I don't like the sandwiches you do,' he said as I started clearing the dinner dishes away. 'Can I have something different tomorrow?' His voice was tired.

'You've been complaining about them every day now.' I continued putting the dishes in the dishwasher. 'I've changed them as much as I can.'

'And I don't like the tea you make.' He stood in the kitchen doorway staring at me as I poured powder into the compartment in the dishwasher, closed the door and turned it on.

'Mum?' one of the girls called from upstairs.

'Look,' I snapped at John, 'if you don't like what I do for you there's one easy cure. You make your own lunches from now on.' I pushed past him and went upstairs.

When I came down, the kitchen bench was covered in crumbs, the butter lay open next to the breadboard and a tin of sandwich spread lay on the draining board, its lid next to the kettle. John had gone to the sitting room. I sighed and put everything away. When I had finished, I went to join him in the sitting room but he wasn't there. I hadn't heard the front door close. Where was he?

'John?' I called. There was no response.

I went upstairs and glanced into our bedroom. John was lying on top of the bed, fully dressed. The room smelled of unwashed clothes. I went to the laundry basket, took the lid off and leant down to pick up a handful of washing.

'Don't!' John snarled from the bed.

'But I've got to wash the clothes,' I replied, 'they're dirty.'

'No, don't do it.' There was a hard edge to his voice. He couldn't be serious. I stared at him. He *was* serious. I shrugged my shoulders, went to the window, opened it a fraction and left the room. I was not looking forward to going to bed that night. Something had to be done, but now was not the time. It would wait until the weekend.

The weekend finally came.

'Right,' I called. 'I've packed the picnic. It's time to get in the car.'

Penny came down the stairs slowly. 'Do we have to?'

'Where are we going?' Emma followed Penny, equally slowly.

'Yes, we have to!' I snapped, then coughed and smiled. 'And it's a surprise. Come on John.' He looked up from his reclining chair in the sitting room. For a moment it looked as if he were going to argue, but when he saw the girls he got out of the chair and joined them.

'Let's go north today,' I said as I drove the car out of our driveway. 'I believe there is a little spot near the Three Pickerels. We'll give it a try.' The girls groaned. John sat numbly in the seat next to me. He resented being forbidden to drive, but I couldn't help that.

The Fen fields were flat, chocolate brown or thinly covered in pale green. A kestrel hovered overhead.

'These compulsory picnics are great, aren't they?' I tried to sound cheerful as I turned towards the Three Pickerels. No one replied. The girls muttered to each other. I could tell that we needed to stop soon before a fight broke out.

I parked the car in a little turning off the road. The gate was new, sturdy and securely locked. It was unlikely any vehicles would want to use it while we were there.

We climbed out of the car, I grabbed the picnic things and we headed for the long straight bank above the dyke. A pocket of reeds swayed gently above the still dark water. The sky was a uniform grey, the clouds smooth and unthreatening. I could feel the tension in my shoulders release as the girls ran on ahead and John walked sombrely beside me.

'We'll stop here!' I shouted to the girls, who turned and started to walk back. An old tree stretched sideways in front of us. Its leaves were large and evergreen, the trunk gnarled and timeless. The lumpy tufts of grass in the field were moist but the ground beneath the tree's branches was dry. I spread out the blanket for us to sit on and laid out the picnic.

'Salad sandwich?' I asked, handing the girls and John a sandwich each. I breathed in the air. Its cool freshness eased my fractious thoughts. I waited until we had finished the picnic and we were on our walk.

I could see the girls walking steadily ahead of us and John and I walked by the dyke, calm and thoughtful in the ghostly quiet of the natural beauty of the scene.

'You know,' I said to John glancing at him, 'I'm very tired these days.'

'You'll have to go to bed earlier,' he said.

'It's not that,' I said, 'It's your night shifts. My sleep is disturbed so often. It's affecting my health.'

I decided against saying how the smell of his dirty clothes was also a deciding factor. He stared ahead.

'Would you mind if we slept in separate beds?'

He did not reply.

'Would you mind sleeping in the spare room from tonight?'

His shoulders drooped. He watched the girls chasing each other along the path ahead.

'I suppose so,' he murmured. My heart clenched. The defeat impregnating his words had hit a raw nerve in both of us. We knew it was the beginning of the end.

It was a bright Saturday afternoon. The girls and I had been to morning school at the private school where I now worked, and I was now trying to sort out the washing from the gym bags they'd dumped by the front door before dashing out to play. Then I heard the swish of John's bike as he sped past the door to park it around the side of the house. I paused, still clutching a pair of the girls' shorts. It was his 40th birthday in a month or so. Life was getting so dull; something had to be done for this special birthday, while he could still appreciate it.

A few moments later John put his key into the lock and swept the door open. A waft of fresh air greeted me as he smiled. His jacket needed a good clean but I had long given up trying to extricate it from him while he was wearing it. I would steal it into the washing when he wasn't looking.

'Welcome home,' I said giving him a kiss. He accepted the kiss absently and said, 'Look what I found on the road. They might be useful.' He pulled a pair of thick red rubber gloves from his jacket pocket.

'Maybe,' I tried to sound supportive. 'You could keep them in the garage with the others.' They went straight back into his pocket. He went into the kitchen and left his plastic lunch container and thermos on the counter and came back to the sitting room to flop into his reclining chair. I finished grabbing the clothes to wash from the girls' bags.

'Cup of tea?' I asked as I went towards the kitchen.

'Yes,' John said as he picked up the newspaper.

As the washing machine spluttered into action, I picked up the tea tray and made for the sitting room. Placing the tray on the table between our chairs, I sat down heavily. The girls were arguing outside the window, but I decided they would have to be closer to murdering each other before I would intervene. I felt too tired anyway.

'You're on nights next week, aren't you?' I asked. John did not reply. He turned over to the next page of the Daily Telegraph. 'Our MP is making himself heard in the Commons.'

I poured milk into the cups and filled them with the tea that had now brewed enough to be the right dark colour for John.

'Your tea,' I said forcibly rattling the cup so he could not avoid it. He folded the newspaper down onto his lap and accepted the cup.

'You're on night shift next week, yes?'

'Yes, what of it?'

'It means you get in at about 6.30 in the morning. I could set the washing to finish then so you could hang out the clothes when you get in, couldn't you?'

'I suppose so.'

'Right, that's decided then. You're hanging out the washing every day.'

John took another sip from his teacup, put it on the table beside him, shook open the newspaper and began to read. That was the first part of his 40th birthday celebration completed.

The next afternoon I got home early from school. John was not back yet. I picked up the phone and dialled our friend Leon's number. Leon and his wife, Annabelle, could be counted on for a bit of fun. I needed to do something to lighten our lives while there was still time.

'Would you come to a party at 6.30 in the morning?' I whispered into the phone just in case John suddenly appeared — something he was doing quite often these days.

'6.30 a.m.! That's a novel idea. What's up?' Leon, constant party instigator, was the most likely candidate to agree to such a wild idea.

'It's John's 40th and he gets back from work at that time.'

'Yeah, we'll come — won't we, Annabelle?' A muffled voice in the background sounded positive.

'I'm not sure how to go about it. What would you serve at that hour in the morning?'

'There's nothing like a champagne breakfast,' Leon said, enthusiastically. With his fleet of sports cars, yacht and luxury lifestyle, he could never understand our financial constraints.

'Er, white bubbly, and what goes with that?'

'I'll hand you over to the wife, she'll have some ideas.'

'Hello?' Annabelle's cheerfulness was apparent in her single word of greeting.

'Hi, it's Sally here. I'm thinking of having a party for John's 40th next week at 6.30 in the morning, but what can I serve, besides white bubbly?'

'Oh, that's easy, just a bit of smoked salmon. That'll go down well. Most of us will have to dash off to work, I guess, so you don't need to go to town. Anything I can do?'

'No, that'll be fine. 6.30 on Thursday then, OK?'

'You're on.'

'Don't say anything to John. It'll be a surprise.' I put the phone down as the key turned in the lock.

'I've posted a letter to the Prime Minister. He's got to understand that without support for our industry, our country cannot survive. I was speaking to the boss only yesterday...' John talked loudly as he went towards the kitchen. He opened the fridge door and took out the lunch box he had prepared earlier. I wondered when he had last washed the box. It must have been several days since he last cleaned it. He'd get food poisoning if he weren't careful. Like a broken record, his voice chugged on without respite.

'Yes, dear,' I murmured, thinking about how I was going to keep the smoked salmon in the fridge without its being taken by him to fill his lunch boxes.

I glanced at the kitchen clock. John paused a moment as he put his box down on the hallway table, reached for his shabby overcoat and took his bicycle clips out of the pocket. He turned to me and with his hand pointing towards me; he took a large breath, opening his mouth to continue.

I quickly butted in. 'Be careful on the roads.'

'Yes, but I just want to say ...'

I opened the front door and shepherded my husband towards the outside.

'Go!' I said in my schoolmarm's commanding tone, but with a conspiratory smile. He smiled back in recognition.

Chapter 31

Thursday morning was bright and sunny. I crawled unwillingly out of bed at 6.00 a.m., dressed and crept downstairs carefully making sure I did not step on the squeaking floorboard so as not to wake the girls, they would have to be woken up soon enough for their school day. As I neared the front door, I heard the swish of John's new bike, his birthday present bought in advance. At least he had got home on time.

'Morning,' I said sleepily. 'Happy birthday' I hugged him. He smelt of sweat. How could I get him to shower before the party? I knew I couldn't, he would soon know something was up.

'I'll get the washing,' John said using his authoritative I'm-a-brilliant-chap tone.

'Thanks,' I said absently, barely giving thought to my usual 'I should think so' response. Once John had taken the basket of wet clothes outside, I went into action, swiftly unwrapping the disguised slivers of smoked salmon and frantically preparing the breakfast feast on the dining room table.

The side-gate rattled. Nelly and Paul, clutching a bottle of wine, walked straight towards John. Still holding a pair of my underpants he turned. He frowned.

'Happy birthday, John!' Paul stepped forward and shook John's free hand. Nelly stepped up quickly after her husband.

'It's a surprise, isn't it?' I grinned.

John's face lit up. They had come to see *him*. He was the centre of attention. Brilliant! He dropped my underpants back into the basket and the three of them came into the dining room. Leon and Annabelle soon made up the modest crowd, bottles of bubbly were cracked open and the party began. John's voice rose in the excitement and while his guests quietly sipped the wine and nibbled the breakfast, he entertained his audience with his strong opinions on the political events of the day, an overabundance of Oscar Wilde quotes and reminiscences of what his father would have said had he still been alive. No one minded - it was too early to have the energy to respond to the highly-charged birthday boy.

When he accidentally knocked Annabelle's glass to the floor and I was frantically trying to sweep up the glass before the girls came down in their bare feet, the party disintegrated as quickly as it had started.

'Must go,' Paul said, giving me a quick hug as I struggled to my feet, dustpan still in hand. He shook John's hand and left, with Nelly in tow. The guests melted and John and I were left alone in the dining room strewn with party debris.

'I must take my medicine,' John disappeared upstairs to bed. I glanced at the clock. In ten minutes I would have to wake the girls. A wave of exhaustion overwhelmed me. I sat down on the nearest chair. A single tear fell down my pale cheek. Why? Inside I felt happy, contented that the party had been successful. Yet, this momentary cloud of dark melancholy invaded my thoughts. I could clear the party things up tonight. I brushed the tear away, forced myself to get up from the chair, and went to wake the girls.

Christmas came and I was determined we would have a good family day — no other relatives (not even Mother-in-law), just the four of us. I had succeeded in demanding that Christmas Day was no longer filled with the tense moaning of his unhappy mother; our girls would have some pleasure in life now that their dad was getting more and more difficult. The morning opening of presents, and Christmas dinner went fairly well, even after the power cut had played havoc with cooking the turkey. We were relaxing in the sitting room and the girls were around the house trying out their new toys. We were waiting for the Queen's speech on TV. Suddenly John stood up.

'Sit down, John!' I giggled.

He did not reply. He remained standing, his shoulders back, his face contorted with emotion. The Queen was about to start her speech on the TV. When the speech finally ended he sat down in his chair.

'Well, thank goodness for that,' I sighed.

'Honour where it is due,' John said. 'Our Sovereign Queen should be given respect.'

'Yeah, but not at home in the sitting room,' I laughed.

John grinned. I was not sure if he had been serious or not.

'She is coming to Ely later on this year,' I said. 'Maybe you would like to see her?'

'I certainly would.' After this, I never heard the end of it. Every conversation was littered with references to Her Majesty. John was in his element.

'Well, at least you'll never be done for treason,' I commented when I had had enough one day. I had my own troubles to deal with. Now Head of Music at a local private school, with some of the boys singing to the Queen when she came, I felt I should make an effort to hear them — even if it was only for the rehearsal.

I had phoned the powers that be only to be given short shrift.

'It is not for the likes of you to attend. No, you may not attend a rehearsal.' What was I to do? If I ignored events, the boys in my classes would think I had snubbed them. I knew I would be able to listen to them on the radio when the Queen came. I decided that was the only workable solution.

'Would you take the girls to see her?' I asked John over our ritual cup of tea.

'Why?' he growled. I bit my lip. I had caught him at the wrong time.

'Because I need to stay at home so I can hear the boy choristers on the radio.'

'Oh,' he slumped into his chair.

'Well get on then,' John snarled, holding out the girls' coats. Wondering if they would be all right with their father when he was in such an impatient mood, I hugged the crying girls and helped them into their coats.

'It will be all right,' I soothed, 'Stay with your dad. There will be a lot of people there.' There will be plenty of people to save them from him if he's too rough, I thought.

I turned the radio on. It crackled loudly. I turned the tuning switch slowly forwards. The sound was hardly any better. I turned it back as far as it would go. The sound was still no good. I opened the front door and turned the switch forwards again. At last I could hear the station I needed. I would have to rush outside when they were on. I left the front door open with the radio blaring as loud as I dared, trying not to annoy the neighbours, and went to finish the washing up and then the remaining paperwork from school. The boys would be singing in five minutes. I put down the file of papers and rushed to the front door. The commentator was talking about the Queen. They would be singing at any moment. I stood still and listened intently.

'Hello!' I jumped. I waved at Mrs Brown, my cleaning lady. Not now! I mimed to her that I was busy. Mrs Brown, a forthright lady with a determination that nearly matched mine, had something very important to say.

The organ began playing.

'I'm sorry Mrs Wilks,' Mrs Brown shouted, to make sure she could be heard above the noise from the radio 'but I have something important to say.'

'Shh! Later?' I asked. The boys' voices were just starting.

She shook her head. 'No, now.'

I turned away from her in a desperate move to listen to the radio. She stepped immediately in from of me. 'I'm sorry; I have to give in my notice now.'

I ignored her at first and then realized the importance of what she had just declared.

'No!' I cried. She could not give notice *now*, now that she was needed more than ever. I was torn. The boys were singing, I must listen to them but Mrs Brown moved closer and folded her arms.

'I won't be in next week. I'm sorry but there is nothing for it. Your husband is very difficult to deal with and I cannot cope with him and the work I have to do. Besides, my Betty is not well and I have to see to her.'

'But —' the boys were well into their music, which had been thoroughly drowned by Mrs Brown's impassioned speech.

'I'll be in on Friday to collect my wages.' She turned tail and as I watched her ample figure waddle down the drive and into the street, the closing notes of the final bars of music faded away on the radio.

I swore. At least John and the girls had probably seen the Queen so the day would not be wasted.

I sat at the desk and began to write on a postcard. 'Wanted, cleaner with a sense of humour ...'

Half an hour later, I could hear the girls crying as they came down the street. Maybe the day had not been a good one after all.

'Daddy was mean,' Penny sobbed as I helped her take off her coat.

'He was so too,' repeated Emma.

'Oh dear!' I looked quizzically at John who was obviously still in a bad mood.

'Well, they wouldn't stand up when the Queen came so I dragged them to their feet. There was nothing else I could do,' John growled, taking his own coat off, hanging it on one of the pegs and climbing the stairs.

I hugged the girls for a moment.

'Well, it's all over now. Maybe you won't have to go to town with Daddy on your own again. Let's go to the kitchen and get a drink and a biscuit.'

I read the letter from my father again. I suddenly yearned to be back in Devonport, Tasmania. I devoured every word, every snippet of news and just for a moment I could imagine I was there with my mum and my dad and my brother, sitting at the kitchen table sharing the gossip of the neighbourhood. Sandy, the Labrador from Number Five in their street had died, Haines' shed had been blown down again, and there was a new ferry crossing from Devonport to Melbourne. Otherwise everything was the same.

I sat back and closed my eyes. At last I had time to think —John had rushed out to see the doctor on a routine visit and the girls were playing with their friends in the garden. Thank goodness someone else had to cope with John's interminable talking. Sometimes I just wished my dad were with us and not thousands of miles away in Australia. The two-year itch niggled at me again. Every two or so years I felt a need to go home, home to Tasmania again, and I wanted to go home now.

I went to the desk in the sitting room, looked for my passport and the travel advertisements I had been saving over the years. It would not hurt to spend time trying to get the paperwork in order. It was always a long drawn-out process, the agony of waiting to get it all sorted usually dampened my desires and I soon settled down into the new life I had created for myself in England. If I just sorted the paperwork out there would be no harm done.

I gasped. At the age of twelve, the girls would have to pay adult fare! Since when was a twelve-year-old girl an adult? Really, these airline firms take the biscuit! That meant that if we ever went as a family we'd have to go this summer.

I heard John's bike rattle past the window.

'I'm home!' John called as he came through the front door. I grinned. At last he was in a good mood!

'Welcome home, John. Was everything all right at the doctor's?'

'It certainly is. I can have my licence back. I can drive again!'

'That's wonderful!' I tried to sound enthusiastic as I hugged him but wondered what I was going to do if he went off with the car when I needed it. I would have to be sure I was in control of the car keys.

'You know we can't afford a second car. We'll have to share.'

John broke free, took off his coat, hung it on the peg and rushed to the desk.

'I'll write to the DVLA now and tell them.'

'But won't the doctor ...?' I sighed. There was no stopping him sometimes. I shrugged my shoulders and let him continue. I would talk about Australia at another time.

The ducks circled on the dark water of Histon's village pond, quacking loudly. John, the girls and I still had our coats on to ward off some of the cold. It was autumn and the air was still damp and cold but this did not stop us from having our picnic; nothing stopped us from having our compulsory picnic.

'Well, you got us here in one piece,' I congratulated John. 'It's really good that you're driving again. It's a pity we can't do something about getting you a car to drive to work.'

'It's okay,' he responded. I'm happy to continue cycling. I'd hate to let Dinah down.'

I bit into my sandwich. Dinah was mentioned quite often these days. 'Dinah?'

'Dinah and I meet up at the crossing now and cycle together from there every day. She's good company. We work together most of the time now, you know. '

I stopped mid-bite into my sandwich and looked my husband in the eye. If it were anyone else in any other relationship, a question mark would hang over such words. An affair? The wife is always the last one to know. I shivered. No, of course not, John was not that sort. He wouldn't.

'You must meet her sometime. I'll get her to ring you,' he said happily.'

'Yes, you must.' I chewed the last remnants of my sandwich slowly. John stood up and went to the water's edge to join the girls while they were feeding the last of their sandwiches to the ducks.

I gathered together the empty lunch boxes on the cloth, shook out the crumbs onto the damp grass, replaced the lids and put the boxes into the picnic basket. I stood up, gathered the edges of the tablecloth together and shook it until it was crumb-free. I folded it as I called, 'Come on.' A drop of rain fell onto my cheek. 'Time to go. It's going to rain.'

The girls ran to the car, John walking jauntily behind them.

'I'll drive a different way home,' he said as he climbed into the driver's seat. 'Buckle up, girls.' He turned on the engine.

'Just let me get the picnic things into the boot first, will you?' I called as I struggled to open the boot and put the basket and cloth inside. I slid into the passenger seat and buckled my seatbelt.

John turned onto the A10 and drove towards home.

'Let's go to Derbyshire for our holidays this year,' he said as he changed up a gear. 'We could go for some walks in the hills every day. The girls would love it.'

'Mm,' said I, deciding not to mention Australia just yet, not while he was driving. As soon as we were home and inside, I would broach the subject.

Once we were safely inside, I asked, 'Would you like to go to Australia? Could we go to Australia for our summer holidays this year?'

'Australia!' He looked at me incredulously. 'Why yes, we must go to Australia. We could stay with your father and I could drive us all around the island, visiting your brother in Hobart on the way. I must write to your father.'

'If we don't go it would cost double to take the girls next year,' I added, speaking to John's back as he went to sit down at the desk. 'Australia here we come' I muttered to myself wondering if it was a wise decision.

Chapter 32

I forced a plastic smile. I was actually floating, floating on a cloud of confusion. I was back in the sitting room at home in Devonport, Tasmania. Everything was familiar yet strange and smaller than I remembered. I wished I could focus better — sleep deprivation and I never did go well together. A whirl of family came and went but all I wanted to do was sleep, but when I finally had a chance to lie down to doze I couldn't, my eyes sprang open, I was wide awake and yet still exhausted.

John and the girls, well they were there somewhere, but they'd have to fend for themselves I decided, at least until I found my feet.

'Dad was in ever such a bad mood,' Emma said, as I sat on the veranda gazing at the gum tree outside the front gate. 'We left him and went into town on our own.'

'Did you dear?' I smiled inanely. Emma harrumphed and went to search for Penny. I could hear John talking non-stop to my father further inside the house. Thank goodness there was someone else to listen to him for a change. The voices suddenly stopped. My heart stopped a beat.

'Enjoying the sun? Getting your daily dose of skin cancer?' John was standing next to me.

'A right ray of sunshine you are yourself, John,' I moaned.

'Ready for Hobart tomorrow?' he continued. 'I'll give your brother a ring to see if everything's ready.'

With that he quickly disappeared into the cool interior of the house.

'Yes. You go ahead. I'll do the packing later tonight,' I sighed not caring if I was speaking to myself or not. Would this exhaustion never leave me?

The following morning, our cases were lined up on the veranda; John had driven the car to the garage in town to be checked for oil and to get petrol. As I hugged my father goodbye a blackbird was singing its heart out in the sunshine that streamed down onto us.

'Got everything, girls?' John asked as they gave their granddad a hug and climbed into the back of the car. I did not care if we had forgotten something; we could always collect it when we came back on our way to the UK.

'You can take the first shift,' I said to John after he had already climbed into the driver's seat. I did not have the energy to argue with him. Besides, it suited me for the moment. We would just have to take the risk.

'Just head south and we'll get to Hobart,' I murmured. At least the roads were clear in this tiny unpopulated island and I might be fully focused by the time we get there, I thought. I settled down in the passenger's seat and closed my eyes. Maybe at last I would be able to relax.

'You must see Port Arthur.' Ray handed me a beer, a gorgeous cold beer. I lifted the glass to my lips. Nectar, sheer nectar. My brother certainly knew how to enjoy life.

'We'll go tomorrow,' John took his glass of lager from Ray and sat down.

'We will?' I smiled. The girls were glued to the TV. An Australian soap was in full swing. I was relieved that it was not 'Neighbours'. No one seemed to watch 'Neighbours' here.

'It's okay,' Ray said quickly, 'yes, we'll go tomorrow. How about we leave at about nine o'clock? That should give us a good day there.'

'Nine it is then.'

The elongated brick façade of the penal colony was bleak and uninhabited. Ray and Elaine parked their car next to a fence adjoining the field in front of the penal settlement. John parked beside them and we climbed out of the car.

'We've seen it all before,' Ray said as he and Elaine climbed out of their car. 'You go on ahead.'

I shivered as the girls ran towards the building.

'Wait for Daddy and I,' I called. The girls slowed a little.

'Of course, once Great Britain could no longer send convicts to America after the War of Independence in 1788, Tasmania was the ideal place to send them.' John pocketed the car keys and straightened the camera that was hanging round his neck. 'The colonies had their uses you know.' He grinned, following the girls. 'You have to understand, one in five of the prisoners was a woman, and there would have been no escape for you if you had committed even the smallest of crimes.'

I gave him a sideways glance. Where did he get all this information? All I could remember vaguely was that it was established in about 1840, which now seemed so recent after living in England where 'old' was not a hundred, but a thousand years of history.

John and I took a number of photos as we approached the long building. We went inside and found a row of tiny, dark and damp cells. Penny leaned in to look inside one of them. Emma stood behind her, craning forward to look too.

John came up behind them. 'Go inside,' he said to Penny. Penny looked up at her father and then inside the dark, damp interior of the cell.

'No,' Penny stepped back, her face pale and anxious. She accidentally trod on Emma's foot.

'Watch out!' yelled Emma.

'Go inside!' John insisted, 'both of you!' He was using that do-as-you-are-told voice that they had learned not to disobey. Looking longingly at me the girls reluctantly stepped into the darkness, the damp stone smelling of years of neglect.

'Pooh, it smells in here,' said Emma her voice trembling and muffled. 'Let us out, Dad.'

'It's horrible! Please, Dad, please let us out. You could go mad in here!' Penny screeched. They both started crying.

John grasped the wooden panelled door. 'It won't hurt you to know what it's like. Your Uncle Jim —' he shouted, pushing the panel door.

'No, don't shut the door on them!' I shrieked, and quickly grabbed John's arm. With a violent shove, he extricated himself from my grip and stepped forward.

'No!' I shouted, grabbing his arm again and pulling hard, 'Don't shut the door!' I swung round in front of him placing myself firmly between John and the cell entrance and glared at him.

John stopped. His eyes wild and bewildered, he reluctantly dropped his hands. Penny and Emma rushed out of the cell, rattling the wooden door in their haste. They stood huddled beside me looking at their dad incredulously.

I put my arms round her girls' shoulders. 'Let's get back to the car, we can go and see the rocks and wild sea that the convicts had to contend with if they wanted to escape.'

We turned and walked smartly to the car. As I sat in the passenger seat I looked at John. He sat next to me, grimly. Then it occurred to me. He had mentioned Uncle Jim. So John knew about Uncle Jim — the same Uncle Jim that Hannah had inadvertently mentioned when we had coffee together so long ago. I needed to know what happened to Uncle Jim and why he was associated with such a ghastly experience as being shut in a dark cell. Maybe he was imprisoned for something. Did John have several criminals in his family? After all, Babs had already told me about his Uncle Matthew Wilks stealing from his company, probably under Eunice's influence at best, or at worst, she was guilty of the crime herself. Was that why he would not tell me about them? One day I would find out.

The waves rose and fell ferociously on the hard rocks at Port Arthur. A cold unforgiving wind lashed at them wildly. I noticed the stones were redder than the black rocks I used to walk on hour after hour when I was a lonely child in Devonport. The sense of isolation brought a rush of the same overwhelming sadness and loneliness I had felt as a teenager all those years ago. I had been young and vulnerable and had felt very much alone. The sun came out for a moment making the spray glisten surreally in the wild isolated landscape.

John and the girls climbed down to the rocks. The girls sat on a strong ledge and dangled their feet over the edge, watching the distant waves as they crashed and split on the shiny rocks. I was happy to survey the scene from a distance. I could see the crashing water breaking through a jagged hollow in the rocks formed by centuries of relentless assault. John climbed further down, right to the thin edge that hung over the tumultuous sea.

'John?' I called. 'Come back. Don't go so close to the edge', but my voice was carried away on the wind. John could not hear me, or he chose not to listen. My heart in my mouth, I stared at the wild sea. Spray splattered over John. One slip and he would be gone. I turned my head away; I could not look. Why did he take such risks? Did he believe he was invincible or was he really fully in command of his movements?

Ray and Elaine walked towards me. 'He's a bit near the edge, isn't he?' Ray said.

'Yes, I know.' I looked pleadingly at my brother.

'John!' he yelled. This time John suddenly turned and looked up at Ray.

'Come on, we're going,' Ray cupped his hands against the wind and shouted. John took one more photo and started towards us. I heaved a sigh of relief.

'It's like having another child, isn't it?' said Ray as we watched John step jauntily over the slippery rocks towards us.

I mused. So, it was not just my imagination. John *was* more than just an eccentric individual; he was slowly degenerating, needing more and more attention like the children I used to teach. Was there any connection with the mysterious Uncle Jim? Maybe he was not a criminal; maybe Uncle Jim's mind went as well? Was this happening to John? Was it hereditary perhaps? I suddenly felt tired. I forced a smile at my brother. I was not going to give in now.

The wind was picking up. I hugged my arms close. 'Come on, girls, time to go.'

Penny and Emma jumped up and ran towards us.

The journey back to Devonport was peaceful, hardly a car to be seen on the single-lane highway. Little towns dotted our trek, towns with familiar names that I half remembered from a carefree childhood: Oatlands, Richmond, Westbury, and Deloraine. Sprawled houses lazed in the winter sun; gum trees lined the roads, wide single main roads had pavements wide enough for an army, shops had large friendly windows. I suddenly missed the crooked narrow streets and buildings of centuries ago in England.

'If you pull over here, John, we can have lunch.' John eased the car next to the pavement. Parking was not an issue here. A postman zoomed past in his tiny vehicle. He had to cover distances that made cycling impossible.

'I haven't had a meat pie for ages — come on, let's go and get some from the shop.' I climbed out of the car and waited until the girls had extricated themselves from their seatbelts and John had locked the car. The girls dashed to the toilets, jostling their way through the narrow entrance. John and I followed. We met as a group outside.

'Meat pies for everyone then?' I grinned. I could taste the steaming beef and onion and pastry that melted in the mouth. I must have been Penny's age when I used to dash to the shop over the road from school to buy my meat pie for lunch.

'I'm not hungry,' John snarled.

'Well, you don't have to eat, but you should. The girls and I are going to have something whatever you say.' John scowled.

We were walking as a group towards the shop that advertised meat pies in large letters on the window.

'I don't want to go back to England,' said Penny, kicking a stone from the pavement into the street. 'Why can't we stay here?'

'You've got school to go to. Besides, your dad and I have our jobs in England. It would not be so easy to get jobs out here.'

'Penny, Emma what would you like to drink?' I hoped John would weaken when he smelt the food. 'Coca Cola for you, John?'

'No, water. Can we go now? We have to get ready to go home tomorrow.' I was painfully aware of this, but would rather not be reminded.

'Just let us have our lunch first,' I said. 'Would you like me to drive now?'

'No!' John snapped. I decided to leave him alone for a bit. Now was not the time to argue with him.

Tired from the journey and with a hundred and one things to do, the evening went swiftly, and I flopped into bed, falling asleep the moment my head hit the pillow. My sleep was restless. I was aware of my husband next to me, twitching with his own anxious dreams. A mysterious figure haunted my dreams, his features very much like John's but his head moving into different surreal shapes. I sat bolt upright. John was sleeping solidly next to me. The light from the streetlight outside the window cast an eerie glow on the blanket. I lay down again, closed my eyes and prayed I would not be haunted by the same nightmare again.

In the early light of the morning, the house was sleeping. The sunlight lit the room cheerily. The ghosts of my nightmare were vanquished. Everything looked brighter, much more hopeful. Everything would be all right. I lay back luxuriating in the few moments I would have to think and rest before leaping out of bed for the day's action-packed scenarios. How I loved the golden glow of the early morning light. The birdsong was joyous and vibrant— far more than I could remember of the dainty calls from the trees near our house in England.

Suddenly John let out a cry. His body convulsed and he screwed himself into a ball. His body shook violently and I could hear the rattle of his teeth and gurgle of saliva slapping his lips. Oh no, not again.

'John!' I cried, leaping out of bed to see that he wasn't choking on his tongue. I was not sure what I could do, even if he was, but thank goodness, he was breathing all right. I hated watching him like this, his body wracked with some hidden disease. It was like an evil possessor taking over his victim, destroying him, piece by piece. How much of the John I knew was being claimed this time?

'Dad?' I called 'Dad!' Every time John had a fit, I panicked. Surely it was about time I was used to this!

'Dad!' I shrieked. I couldn't help myself. 'John's having a fit. Can you call the doctor?' I heard the thump of my father's feet as he hurriedly leapt out of bed.

By the time the doctor came we were all crowded round the bed. Penny and Emma half awake, their cheeks pale, my dad frowning, not certain where to look or what to do with his hands. The doctor sat on the edge of the bed and looked at John who by now had finished thrashing about. John was lying still, confused. He stared at the stranger next to him, puzzled.

'Yes, a fit in the temporal lobe area,' the doctor murmured. I looked quizzically at Dr Hopkins, the doctor I had known since childhood. He had not grown any older. His smooth polished skin and bright dark eyes were just the same. I blushed, wondering if he remembered that terrible visit when I had had a fever. He had kicked the full potty that was under the bed and drenched his shoes with urine. I grimaced momentarily. He stood up unaware of my discomfort.

I blurted, 'What can we do? We're leaving to go back to England this afternoon?' I asked.

'He'll be all right.' He took out a pad from his bag and started writing. 'I'll write you a note to take with you and give you some Valium to give him if he needs it.'

I wanted to ask how I would know if he needed it. There was never any warning when John had one of his turns. Besides, if he were in a bad mood, he certainly would not take anything from me. I smiled weakly, accepted the note and the Valium and watched Dad show him the way out.

'Well, good on you, John, nothing like a bit of excitement before we set off.' I tried to make my sarcasm sound cheerful in front of the girls.

He looked puzzled.

'How do you feel now?'

'I'm all right,' he said, stepping out of bed. 'Off you go girls; I'm going to get dressed.'

'So when should you have your next dose?' I asked. John shrugged.

'Soon we'll be in Hong Kong. Well, if I calculate in twenty-four-hour slots no matter whether it's day or night on whichever side of the world we are ...' I hated being responsible for his medication like this — what if I got it wrong? What if he had another fit? When we get home, I thought, I'll take John straight to the GP, hand him all the medication and let the GP work it out from there. Yes, that was the solution. I felt better.

Chapter 33

Our journey by plane to Melbourne was uneventful. We finally found our places on the plane that was taking us to England and settled ourselves for the long journey. I looked around at the half-sleeping, half-dozing people propped uneasily in their seats. One very large woman in the aisle seat on the other side of the plane was snoring heavily.

I nudged John. 'I hope I don't snore like that.' John was fiddling with his camera and did not answer. Did that mean that I did snore or that he was not interested?

'You really can be annoying sometimes,' I quipped.

8'I don't know *what* you are talking about!' John replied and I knew that he was telling the truth this time. What was the truth about Uncle Jim? Would he tell me some day? And there was Dinah. He was returning to his work at the factory and to Dinah. Was he telling the truth about his new friendship with Dinah though? How could I find out? I could hardly follow him — I had to be at work and there were so many things to keep me busy in the house. I settled down further into my seat. I would try to doze at least — I needed the rest.

Finally back home in England the routine settled down again. The following Saturday afternoon the phone rang.

'Hello?' I wasn't expecting anyone to call.

'Is that Sally?' a deep female voice asked.

'Er, yes.' Who could it be?

'It's Dinah Smith here. John told me to call you.'

'Oh.' Now what was I supposed to do? If they were having an affair did I really want to speak to her? But what if they weren't? There was only one sure way of finding out; I would have to meet her. Taking a deep breath, I said, 'Why not come over for a cup of tea this afternoon?'

'All right,' she said, her voice tinged with uncertainty.

At four o'clock on the dot, a figure in reflective bike wear swung into our drive. She leaned her bike against the side of the house and rang the doorbell.

The children were playing happily outside in the garden. No doubt if they had a problem they would soon come in and let me know. I went to the front door. Well, at least there was not an hourglass silhouette behind the glass in the door. I took in a deep breath and opened the door. I let out my breath quickly. This was no glamour girl in front of me. Her face was weathered, without make up, her hair cut in a pudding basin style and her clothes shabby and factory-worn.

'I'm sorry,' she said, 'but John insisted.'

'That's all right, welcome.' I stepped back and let her in. 'Come and sit down while I make the tea.'

'I'm afraid I've got my work clothes on,' she said looking at our sofa as though it were too good for her to sit on.

'John's always sitting down with his work clothes, so I wouldn't worry about that. I'll be back in a minute,' I said over my shoulder as I went to the kitchen.

I soon returned with the tea tray and Dinah was sitting in exactly the same position as when I had left her.

'Mum?' Penny called loudly from the hall. 'Have you got a hammer and nails? We've accidentally pulled off the trellis from the wall.'

'You'll have to wait until your father is ready. I am no good with DIY,' I shouted back. I bit my lip. John would be furious. He hated accidents. I would just have to wait until he was in the right mood to tell him.

'I'll have a go if you like,' Dinah stood up. She gave me a questioning glance. I nodded and she went and joined Penny and Emma.

'Penny,' I heard her say as they went towards the back door, 'can you show me where your dad keeps his tools?'

I shrugged. It was getting harder to imagine Dinah having an affair with John.

'Do you mind if I use your bathroom?' Dinah came back inside. I went to meet her.

'Job done.' She smiled.

I gestured. 'It's the first on your left,' I grinned, 'Thank you *so* much for fixing the trellis. John would have been furious and these days I am not sure if he would have fixed it properly.'

I went to the sitting room to collect the teacups. I heard the flush of the toilet and the door slam as Dinah joined me.

'He's getting to be a bit of a challenge these days, isn't he?'

'You could say that again!' I grinned. At last there was someone who understood.

'He comes over quite often when you're at work. If any of my boys are off school he plays cards with them. We are used to him now, so if any time you want me to John-sit...' She left the sentence unfinished, checking to see if I were agreeable to her suggestion.

'Oh, yes please. I'm going on a conference for work in a fortnight. The girls are staying with friends, but I was a bit worried about what John would get up to while I was away. Could he stay with you then?'

'No problem. My husband and the boys will enjoy the company. No doubt he will enjoy helping me look after my menagerie.'

'Your menagerie?'

'Yes I have four guinea pigs, three cockatiels, six budgerigars, ten species of fish, a dog, a cat, a duckling and a tame crow.'

'Wow, I don't know how you have time for it all.'

'I don't really, but it keeps me busy. Word has got around that I love animals so the boys and their friends keep bringing me baby birds that have fallen out of their nests. The crow has become part of the family. They found the duckling wandering alone along the path — no sign of her mother or the other ducklings.'

'John always wanted to be a farmer, so I think he will be in his element.'

John's stay with the Smiths was a great success, largely due to Dinah's easy-going manner and her people-managing skills.

'He only wanted an envelope and a stamp at three in the morning,' she giggled when she came on her next visit to ours. 'And when he brought a huge mirror home he had collected from the rubbish tip and decided he was going to put it up with the hammer and saw he had salvaged from the tip, I decided he wouldn't.'

We both laughed. I remembered the ghastly afternoon he had tried to take a hammer to our hot water tank — another tussle I had fortunately won.

'I really appreciate what you've done. If there is any way I can repay you?'

'It's all right, we enjoy having him.' She stood up. 'We had fun trying to teach the duck to swim in our bath. We should release it soon. Perhaps you would like to come and see us do it?'

'I'd love to.'

The afternoon of the duck release came. The whole family climbed into the car and I drove to the Smiths' house in the next village. John looked shabby even though he had tried to dress for the occasion. I had been unable to separate him from his clothes to get them cleaned and his shaving was incomplete. An old hat jammed on his head failed to cover the extra whiskers that surrounded his face, but he was happy, so what else mattered?

Dinah got a cardboard box ready. The duck was waddling happily in the garden, the cat eyeing it jealously from the window inside. The girls ran to catch the duck but it swiftly half flew and half waddled under the foliage by the pond. The girls made another dive into the bushes, the duck quacked raucously, and the girls came out empty handed.

Dinah's husband opened the door and, grabbing the opportunity, the cat shot outside.

'I'll get the duck, shall I?' said Dinah.

'No, I will,' John said, as he lumbered heavily towards the pond. The cat ran across the lawn straight in front of John and in one glorious movement he fell straight into the pond. The duck quacked loudly and sped off towards the back of the garden. John stood up slowly, spluttering, water dripping off his saturated clothes.

'No,' laughed Dinah, '*I'll* get the duck.' We were all laughing so much we could only watch her calmly approach the evasive bird and whistle to it gently as she leaned down to put her hands firmly round its tiny wings, carry it to the front of the garden and put it securely into the box.

'Len's got some clothes you can change into, John,' she said, as she watched John stagger up the garden path, his soggy clothes clinging to him. 'Len, can you go and get some clothes for John?'

'We'll drive to the river at Ely,' John announced as we climbed into the car. Len's clothes sagged around his slim frame, but at least they were clean.

'Yes,' said Dinah, 'that would be as a good a place as any.'

A dull sky greeted us when we arrived at the bank of the Great Ouse. We parked very close to the bank and we all climbed out of the car, looking forward to this special occasion when the duck would have its first swim in open water. The river was dark and cool but there were hardly any other ducks or geese to molest it.

'I'm a bit worried,' said Dinah as she placed the box on the damp grass. 'He had not quite got the hang of swimming in the bath. Perhaps we should find somewhere where it is very shallow?'

I looked down at the river. It was so deep I couldn't see the bottom.

'Yes —' I was about to suggest we went elsewhere when John suddenly bent down, opened the box, grabbed the bewildered duck, strode to the water's edge and flung the duck high in the air towards the centre of the river.

'John!' Dinah and I screeched simultaneously.

'Dad,' the girls moaned.

'It *will* swim,' he announced. We watched with bated breath as the little duck scrabbled on and under the water.

Dinah was taking her jumper off, ready to rescue the poor thing, when, quacking loudly, the duck flapped its little wings and struggled wildly until it finally managed to keep some of its body above water as it scrabbled at great speed towards the other bank. Then, in a split second, it sat serenely on the water, its little feet paddling rhythmically.

'Well, thank goodness for that,' I sighed.

'That was lucky,' said Dinah.

John ignored us and walked towards the bridge.

'John,' I called. 'Wait for us.'

Dinah pulled her jumper back on hurriedly and put the box back in the car while the girls and I tried to catch up with John before he created more mischief.

The following Saturday it was Emma's birthday.

'What would you like to do for your birthday, Emma?' I asked as she was preparing for bed one night.

'I'd love to go in a rowing boat, one like my best friend's at school,' she said, reaching for her toothbrush. 'And I would like Granny to come too.' My face fell for a moment, but I quickly assumed a smile and said, 'We'll see what I can do.' I gave her a peck on the cheek and went downstairs to the phone. I asked Babs if she knew where we could hire a rowing boat locally.

The day arrived.

Eunice arrived early. 'My friend Deborah will call for me at 4.00 p.m.,' she said walking smartly inside. 'Where is Emma?'

'She'll be down in a minute,' I smiled falsely. Fortunately I had had a good night's sleep so I was ready to deal with John's mother.

We set off, Eunice sitting glumly next to me, John and the girls in the back.

We drove into a large car park. There were only two other cars there.

'Right,' said John as I pulled on the handbrake, 'everyone out. Let's go. There must be some reason for all those swimming lessons you girls have.'

'But we haven't brought our swimming suits,' Emma said.

'With or without the swimsuits, we're going to get into some rowing boats and muck about on the water. All right?'

'Ooh, yes please,' Emma said scrambling out of the car quickly.

'Wait for me!' said Penny as she undid her seat belt and leaped out too. John slid across the seat and out into the car park.

'I'll watch from the shore,' Granny said, as she waited for John to open the car door for her.

A young boy came towards us.

'Got yer tickets?' he asked. I took out my purse and paid for our tickets. The boy led us through to the lakeside.

'There they are,' he said, as he pointed to a row of boats tied loosely to a short jetty.

I noticed there were no life jackets. I paused. The girls and John were walking to their boats. I grimaced and persuaded myself — I used to play in a rowing boat when I was a youngster and I had not worn a life jacket then, so the girls should be all right this time.

We had four small rowing boats between us. As I pulled on my oars, I could feel something pulling. I looked down and the lake was full of weeds. Slowly we pulled on the oars until we formed a little group stretching towards the centre of the lake. The water was dark and deep and we were enjoying ourselves. I was taking my time, hugging the shoreline. The girls and John were much further out. I stopped and gazed at the scene. I thought fondly of the time we had gone to Flatford Mill — Constable country — as a courting couple. John had taken the oars that time and I remembered admiring his strength and stamina. He was some fit young man.

There was a splash. Our younger daughter cried out. She had fallen in, her boat had overturned. What about the weeds? She could get caught up in them. This was how people drowned. I was petrified.

'Emma, hold on, we're coming!' I shouted to her.

John was the closest boat to her. He sat in his rowing boat, not moving.

'John,' I yelled at him. 'Didn't you see your daughter fall in?'

'Yes,' he said coldly, as if it was a matter of fact, nothing to do with him.

'John. *Do* something. She needs our help. For goodness sake, row out to her!' He ignored my pleas and remained immobile, hardly aware of his younger daughter's plight. I was beside myself. I had to stop myself from physically attacking the man to bring him to his senses and probably upturning his boat as well. I looked over to Emma.

I shouted to Emma again. 'Hold on! You'll be all right. We'll come and get you.' She had heard me and had not panicked. I was so relieved. But she was not yet out of danger. She could not swim to shore; the weeds would weigh her down.

John still did nothing. John's mother had stood up to see what the commotion was. I shouted to John 'Row out to her John!' but still John did not react.

I stared at Emma in desperation. Maybe I could wade and then swim out to her if John was not going to do anything. I could have waded or swum to John and tried to grab his oars and force him to row but I knew that he would not let go. We would end up fighting over the oars and our daughter would drown. I don't know what I thought I was going to do but it was obvious that John was not going to help. If I tried to swim to her I would not be able to make it through all of those weeds. I was frantic. John's mother was standing on the edge of the shore stretching up to see what was happening. I shouted at John again.

'John, row out to her. You must row out to her and help her.' Finally he turned to face me. He gradually realized that something was up and he needed to act. Finally he pulled on the oars and rowed towards the frightened child. She grabbed hold of her dad's boat and clambered in. I heaved a sigh of relief.

It was shocking enough to see our daughter get into difficulty but just as shocking was to discover that John could have easily let her drown. His daughter whom he loved so dearly could easily have been killed and he seemed as if this would have had no effect on his feelings.

I realized then that John's condition was getting very serious. John could not be trusted to behave instinctively or to respond to situations in a normal way.

Our journey home was gloomy. Eunice's tenseness soured the atmosphere in the car. After her tirade at John, mainly about how silly the whole idea had been, how cold she had been, how annoyed she was with Emma for falling in and for the time she had to wait while I towelled Emma down and changed her clothes, the car assumed an air of stifled silence.

Chapter 34

One Friday afternoon just after we had got back from school, the phone rang.

'This is Harriet Bendall.' My stomach tightened. What bombshell was she going to drop now? 'It is important you both see the psychologist for our report. I have made an appointment for you two tomorrow at 4.00 p.m., at the Health Centre. Be there!'

'B-but —' I stuttered. The phone clicked and was silent. What was I going to do? I had to get the girls looked after, take off the last lesson at school and persuade John to turn up. I picked up the phone and dialled frantically.

'We have to visit another doctor,' I said to John as I persuaded him to get into the car. His factory had been very accommodating and Fiona, a seasoned teacher, had agreed to do my cover. John sat in the passenger seat smiling.

'So, another doctor, eh?' He pulled his shoulders back. He would be the centre of attention. 'Of course a doctor is the only person who buries his mistakes,' he laughed.

We arrived at the Health Centre and were shown into Room Three. I was relieved that there was no sign screaming of psychiatrists or psychologists. I was sure John would have run a mile if he had seen any of these.

'I'm Doctor Nielson,' said a tall slim man with straight black hair plastered flat over his forehead, stretching a large hand towards us. We shook his hand in turn and sat down.

'I'm sorry I missed you for the last two appointments.'

'But —' I was about to protest that I knew nothing about the appointments when the doctor held up a warning hand to stop me. I glanced at John who blushed but grimly set his lips together and looked straight ahead. I wondered. Dinah had hinted that John had a knack of avoiding what he did not want to do and that he might have gone so far as to hide certain letters in the mail. Now I was sure that was what he had done.

'Do you mind if I ask you some questions, John?' asked Dr Nielson.

'I'd be delighted,' John grinned. He loved answering questions. He nearly always knew what the answers were, no matter what information was required. Len had often moaned about John when we played Trivial Pursuit. John always knew the answers, except that lately he was blurting them out, ruining any sense of competition.

'What is the date today?' was the first of a barrage of easy questions. John answered them correctly and I sat smugly beside him. I could answer them too, so I was not mad either.

'Who is the Prime Minister?' I knew the answer to that one.

'Who's the Chancellor of the Exchequer?' Mmm. I could manage that one too.

'Who is the Foreign Secretary?' Who is it? I wondered. I felt I should have known, but this was the least of my worries at this time.

John answered immediately and correctly. This was John's expertise. He knew who was who in the government, he knew exactly the situation in the world outside, but if you asked him how *I* felt? At this stage in our relationship it seemed beyond his comprehension, or most likely he may have understood, but he was unable to express himself or to respond. He sensed that things were not right because he was being questioned by so many different doctors so all his concentration was focused on his own survival. I frowned. These questions were not going to demonstrate what was wrong. If the doctor keeps asking this kind of question, I thought, John is going to score better than the sanest of people.

Then came some tricky questions:

'Who is the Minister for Trade in the Opposition?' I sat numbly beside John. I had no idea. John answered the question immediately and the psychologist nodded. I squirmed in my seat. Maybe I was the one that was losing it.

'Thank you,' Dr Nielson said finally. 'Now, John, would you mind if I had a word with your wife alone?' John magnanimously agreed and shot out of the room. I gulped and quickly drew in a large breath. Did this mean I was really done for?

'Can you give me some more information about John?' I let out my breath and relaxed.

'What would you like to know?'

'Can you tell me if his problem came on suddenly or was it a slow progression?'

'It came on very slowly.'

'Is his personality changing completely or is it an exaggeration of the personality he has always had?'

The questions continued and I did my best to answer them truthfully and accurately.

The doctor asked me many more questions that were subtle and searching and I answered as best as I could, but I could not see that this would lead to any definite conclusion. Fortunately I was not a psychologist so he might have found out a lot more and perhaps we would get to the bottom of John's troubles and they would be able to help him.

At the end of the consultation I thanked the doctor and went out of the room to find John talking loudly to the receptionist.

We sat in silence as I drove home. We waited for the results of this meeting. Maybe now the doctors and the Social Services could do something at last.

Nothing happened.

With the tenacity of a drowning man, John clung to his daily newspaper. He insisted on reading it cover to cover and now took to solving the crossword. It was as if he knew his mind was going, but he was refusing to accept it. He was all right as long as he understood the newspaper, could remember its contents and could complete the crossword.

One Sunday afternoon John had just completed the crossword in the paper, the girls were playing outside and I brought in the tea try. At last we could relax. John sat in his chair, frowning.

'Is anything the matter?' I asked. He did not reply. 'Are you having trouble?'

He put his head in his hands. 'I'm confused. I don't know.'

'I know,' I went over to him and put my hand on his. I was curious. 'What does it feel like?'

'I feel as if —' he paused, his frown deepening. 'It feels as if my brain is scrambled,' he said.

I was shocked. How awful, not only to know that your brain is failing you, but also to be aware of it at the same time.

'It might be a good idea to keep a diary. I'll get you one. Now, would you like a cup of tea?'

That night I heard movement on the landing. I turned and looked at my clock. It was three in the morning. I grabbed my dressing gown and crept to my door. I could hear gentle shuffling, definitely not the sound of a burglar trying to move silently. I heard fingers scrabbling at something. I opened my door an inch.

John was in his pyjamas scrabbling at the door at the top of the stairs.

'What are you doing, John?' I asked.

'Going to work,' he replied.

'But it's the middle of the night. You don't have to get up for another four hours. Go back to sleep.'

When I woke up the next morning and went to check John he was lying in bed asleep as I had hoped but there was a distinct smell of urine. John had wet the bed. I asked him to get out of bed, changed the sheets and gave him clean pyjamas.

'Have a shower before you get dressed, John,' I said trying to disguise the annoyance I felt.

One Sunday afternoon we were having our usual compulsory picnic. We had finished eating and were coming back from a short walk, admiring the river and watching a bright kingfisher flashing to and from its nest in the bank of the river. An elderly lady was standing admiring the bird too. As we walked past, John broke away from the family group.

'You'll want to go for a walk,' he said to the lady and put his hand firmly under her arm.

'But —' the lady protested.

'John!' I called. 'Come on, we're going home. Girls,' I said, 'get in the car.' Then I turned to John again. He was still guiding the lady on a walk that she had had no intention of taking. She looked at me despairingly.

'John!' I shouted, 'Leave the lady alone. Come here!'

John ignored me. This was getting serious.

'Look, John,' I screamed, 'I'm going to drive off now. If you don't come *now* I'll leave you behind.'

He hesitated but did not leave the lady's side.

I sighed and walked towards him. I knew that I did not have the strength to manhandle him and force him back to the car. What would I do if he still did not come? I couldn't bear to think about it.

'I'm terribly sorry,' I said to the lady. I put my hand on John's arm. 'Now come home this instant!' I hissed in John's ear using my bossy teacher tone. He slowly let go of the lady and walked beside me as I marched him to the car.

That was the last of our picnics.

I arrived home from school the next Thursday to find the phone pad filled with his writing.

I read his firm angular writing, the writing unevenly distributed across the lines.

'Remember, your school hall cost £4,000,000 to keep it standing and the Luftwaffe were not allowed to bomb it, and the RAF were not today allowed to bomb it because it's a landmark. Stop the loft overflowing by switching off your immersion heater; you had a hot bath didn't you. The USAF know where Ely Cathedral is because they fly round it like St Paul's Cathedral is unusual but you can see it from Greenwich observatory. Canary Wharf cost you millions and you can see it when you go to see your secret friends in Wales. The RAF know I exist because it's on my birth certificate 4 July 1046 sergeant RAF.'

Poor John, I thought. What could I do to help him?

One day the following week, I was in before John. The girls had rushed upstairs to change so they could get down into the sitting room in time to see their favourite TV programme before doing their homework. The phone rang.

'Hello?'

'Hello, this is Guy Buchanan, John's boss.'

'Yes?'

'Is John there or can you speak?'

'He's not home yet. Why, what's the matter?'

'I'm afraid there was an incident again today.'

'Again?'

'Yes, he's having a bit of trouble getting on with his workmates. Last week I had to give him a first warning when he refused to work with one of his colleagues.'

317

'Oh.' I wasn't surprised, but what could I do?

'And today he threw an ash tray at a woman who was having a cigarette in the smoking area.'

'Oh, I am sorry. Is there anything I can do?'

'Not really, but I thought I should warn you that if anything else happens I might have to let him go.'

'Oh,' my shoulders drooped. 'Thank you for letting me know.' I sat down and sighed. Now what?

The next day he hit a woman and had to come home early. She had joked about the royal family. John lost his job at the factory.

He cycled round the village and to and from Ely like a man searching for something special, something he had lost and something that he was insistent on searching for, no matter what words of help and advice anyone had to offer.

As he passed the villagers, they turned and muttered amongst themselves. More and more times I decided he was in no fit state to come shopping with me or to an evening event. I could never be sure what he would do.

'I have an appointment with the doctor at the Health Centre,' he called proudly as he sped off on his bicycle one Thursday just before the girls and I were leaving for school. I sighed. At least I knew where he would be today.

We struggled through the next few months.

One Friday John had left me yet another of his wordy notes.

'My employer complained to my wife who is Head of Music at her school (a thrice graduate of music) who has had me in hospital at Cambridge because of my behaviour is not normal for a normal adults — I have not been to work since 3 July and been on so called sick leave until 11 September. My licence revoked by my doctor. My wife drives. Bad brakes create accidents.'

There was no denying it. The threats that Babs had warned me about were creeping in.

Chapter 35

The next day the doorbell rang. I opened the door to find Mildred looking more contrite than I had ever seen her.

'Are you busy?' she asked.

'No.' For Mildred, I was never busy. Her charming smile and motherliness always helped to ease the stress I was feeling. 'Come in.'

'It's about John,' she said as she stepped over the threshold.

I sighed. It was bound to be about John. 'What has he been up to now?' I asked.

'I saw him cycling off just now so I thought I should come and tell you. Where are the girls?'

'They're visiting a friend who lives around the corner,' I said.

'Well,' she said, pushing out her ample chest, 'he came to my place when I had my niece visiting on Monday. My niece is only fourteen years old and he insisted on talking most inappropriately to her.' She bent her head and whispered, 'He was talking about sex.' She blushed and hung her head.

'He did? I *am* sorry. I have no control over him.'

What more could I say? I made a mental note to mention this at our joint appointment at the doctor's the following week.

As Mildred walked slowly down the drive, a large Mercedes pulled up. Uncle Matthew climbed out of the driver's seat and walked swiftly towards me.

'I was on my way to Cambridge when I thought I'd pop in for a cup of tea, okay?' He grinned. My heart missed a beat — he had that same grin of John's that always caught me unawares.

He hugged me. 'Oh,' he said turning to look at his car. 'Don't worry about that. It's the firm's car. I'm delivering it for them.'

'Oh,' I blushed, 'do come in.' I stepped back and closed the door behind him.

'So,' he said pushing the papers off a chair and sitting down, 'how are you?' I bit my lip. His voice was smooth and sympathetic. I was not going to cry. Every time anyone had been sympathetic to me lately I had burst into tears. I was not going to do that now.

'All right,' I gulped.

He sat forward. 'I thought I should tell you I'm getting some weird letters from John these days. They ramble on and on and do not always make sense. Can I do anything?'

'No, no, he's seeing the doctors. I don't know what else we can do.'

'Well, girl,' he patted my hand, 'I'm always here if you need me.' He handed me his card, which I put in my pocket. 'You know, I was very much in love with his mother once.'

I smiled weakly, finding it hard to imagine.

He leaned back in his chair. 'She was very good-looking in her youth. I would have done anything for her – well, I did.' He blushed and cleared his throat.

I looked at him directly. 'Do you think she was the one who stole money from your firm?' I blushed too; maybe I was going too far.

322

He looked at his feet and paused.

'Maybe, but it was so long ago. The crime has been punished so it would do no good to upset everyone again.' He looked straight into my eyes. I nodded.

He sighed. 'I understood why she stopped seeing me and married Walter when I got into trouble. She is very sensitive you know.'

I smiled. I could see that there was no use in trying to persuade him otherwise.

'You will phone me if I can help?' he asked.

I blinked and smiled. 'Thank you,' I said, and bent my head as I gathered up the teacups. Uncle Matthew was already at the front door.

'Must go, they'll be wondering where I am.' I opened the door and he swept out, gave me a wave, stepped into his car and sped off. I shut the door, went into the sitting room and burst into tears.

Work conferences took on a new role. No longer were they a nuisance that interfered in family life, they were a pleasant respite from what was going on at home. Whenever the girls wanted to stay over at a friend's, join a new afternoon club or go camping, they were always delighted when I agreed immediately.

One of the first work conferences I had attended was held in Cambridge. I had sat at the back of the room and joked about the difference between what we were being told and reality when the chap next to me had burst into laughter. I had put my finger to my lips and glared at him. He had winked back. Charlie and I were friends from that moment. Fortunately he was married and had features that reminded me of my worst enemy at school, so he was bound to be no more than a friend. I knew I would not have the troubles Dennis Parker had raised, thank goodness.

Soon after the conference, Charlie had invited the whole family for the weekend to meet his wife, Pippa and his two children. John had been on his best behaviour and we had invited them back and over the years we had visited back and forth many times.

'We're going to stay with Charlie and Pippa for a few days,' I said to John one afternoon as we sat down to our daily cup of tea.

'Who? Who are they?' he snapped. 'I've never heard of them!'

'Yes, you have,' I replied. 'We've been there many other times. Don't you remember?' He scowled into his teacup.

After a tortuous journey we finally arrived. I hugged Pippa. The girls chatted with their children. Oh, it was such a relief to have someone else helping me deal with the family. I relaxed.

'Let's go for a walk to the park,' suggested Charlie. The day was sunny and warm. It seemed like a very good idea.

'We have only a short stretch of the busy main road to cross and we're there,' Pippa said.

We walked out of their large gated house, turned right into the path adjoining the main road and stood on the edge of the pavement waiting for the traffic to ease. Without warning, John walked straight out into the traffic. Cars screeched to a halt, horns blared and, miraculously, John ended up safely on the other side.

'John!' the adults screeched in unison. Penny and Emma glared at their father. John was oblivious.

'Stay there!' I shouted as we waited until the stalled cars had restarted their motors and the traffic had calmed down.

'I say,' said Charlie, 'he's a bit dangerous, don't you think?' Yes he was dangerous, I thought, but what could I do about it? I hung my head.

The afternoon got worse. When we returned to the house John harangued the family with his rambling thoughts when we returned from our visit to the park.

'Now listen, John.' Charlie had had enough. 'Listen, John,' he repeated pointedly, 'you're being a bore.'

I grinned. At last someone was getting John to face up to the fact that there were other people to consider.

Charlie stared straight into John's eyes. 'Let someone else have a chance to speak.' John blinked. But Charlie's message got through and from that moment our time with this lovely family was ruled by Charlie keeping John in check. It was hard work, but I felt a strong sense of relief. I was no longer alone. There were other people who understood how I felt and were willing to try to help us as much as they could.

After we returned home, I was changing his bed again when I spied his diary left open next to his bed. I no longer felt guilty about reading his diary. It was important that I tried to understand what he was thinking and tried to pre-empt anything he might do.

I read:

'Sally and girls got a letter today from Charlie and Philippa inviting the three sans John to theirs for half term holiday yes and John go to Dinah's that time and feed cats Sally could bring home a book John bought in Australia which Charlie has had for two years, as a native of the UK can understand why the book is not allowed in Britain. All the adults Sally and John met down under were reading this book John bought for $9 in 1988 and brought home. Prime Minister Thatcher caused £m to be spent in stopping the book in Britain and why Thatcher could do a deal with Soviet Michael Gorbachev in London.'

The phone rang:

'I thought you ought to know, John is threatening to do something to your car,' Dinah said.

'That's nothing new,' I said, trying to laugh it off.

'No, I think you ought to be careful.'

What could I do? I was no car mechanic. I had no idea what he could do to the car to stop me using it. Besides, in my heart of hearts I sensed that even though John was losing his mind, there was still that inner core of him that would prevent him for doing anything to endanger our lives, well, not deliberately.

In moments of quiet when we were talking there were other clues that life for us could be getting more dangerous. We were watching a TV program about the Second World War and the atom bomb.

I asked John, 'What if an atomic bomb was dropped on us? What would you do?'

'I'd kill you and the girls and then myself,' John said evenly.

I laughed. 'Don't we get a say in it?'

He did not respond. In his mind it was the first and only thing to do. I gave him a sideways glance. It was most unlikely that a bomb would be dropped on us, so there was no real need to worry ... was there?

Sometime later, I recalled how John had described the effect of the unexpected death of his father. His father had apparently had no more than a cold. He had continued working and only come home for a rest. IIe had died in the night. It was a shock for the whole family.

'When I learned that my father had died I had a nightmare that night. I imagined a huge atomic bomb going off,' John had said. Sometime later I realized that we were indeed in great danger. If John had had a shock, he could easily have dreamt of an atomic bomb exploding again. He would have then killed us. In his mind he would be doing something right and noble. We would not have any say in it. But I did not let myself think of this at the time. I was busy surviving, trying to keep John on the straight and narrow, trying to prevent him from upsetting too many people or creating havoc in the household.

One day I was at the sink thinking about our lot. It's like living with a madman, I thought. Then it dawned on me that it was not just *like* living with a madman, he had in fact turned the corner and we *were* living with a madman.

I *really* had to have some help and have it soon.

John had the uncanny knack of sounding perfectly all right, especially in front of important people or people who mattered when evaluation of his mental condition was concerned. I had learned to let him talk non-stop about what the papers said and to continue with our lives as though his input did not interfere at all.

He often busied himself with the neighbours, much to their consternation. No amount of persuasion would encourage him to desist from doing this. His diary entry at the time reads:

'19 May 92 I observed new next door neighbour has rotary clothes line called to speak to them at no 19 no answer at door bell at 9 am so I wrote to them a letter advising the hazard to their young children and their clothes line possible causing serious injury to child – left note of same with Sally Adults know better but they have to be warned logic a gun kills so does a clothes line with a young child equally not allow child to wander across a road'

One Friday, I was driving us to our next doctor's appointment when he said, 'You turn left here.'

I took in a deep breath, closed my lips tight, blocked my mind to his command and turned right — the way we needed to go. He said nothing. I let out my breath quickly. Thank goodness he did not get angry when I ignored his command this time.

The doctor hummed and hawed and sounded sympathetic, but he did nothing. I drove home tight-lipped. I had to do something.

'Penny and Emma, can you come here?' I called to the girls when John had gone outside to do some digging. 'I have something important to discuss.'

Their faces were serious at they stood in front of me.

'You know your dad is becoming more difficult these days?' They nodded slowly, their little faces very serious.

'I need to know ...' I put my arms around them, 'I need to know what you think.' They huddled together and were silent. I persisted. 'I think your dad is becoming too dangerous for us. I think he needs to be under the doctors' care, possibly in a hospital. I'm going to try to get them to do this. What do you think?'

Penny nodded silently, tears streaming down her face.

Emma looked at me grimly. 'I suppose you have to do what you have to do.' She broke free from my arms and ran to her room.

Chapter 36

At our next meeting with our doctor there were three doctors sitting behind a large desk. After they had seen us both, the leading doctor asked to see me alone. A nurse was looking after John. 'The type of illness John has may be hereditary although we are not certain about this, but I see in our files that you gave your mother-in-law's maiden name as Cox. We have a Jim Cox on our files. He was a farmer from Holywell, institutionalized by his family and died some years later. Any relation?'

'That must be Uncle Jim!' I blurted. So, there is *madness* in the family. Oh please, not John too.

'Ah,' he nodded. 'We think your husband has Pick's disease.' His voice was gentle, almost apologetic. 'I'm afraid we cannot be certain of the diagnosis but it seems to be most likely that this is the disease he has.'

I had never heard of Pick's disease. It had an unfamiliar sound to it. If John just had epilepsy, then everyone would know what I was talking about — but 'Pick's disease'? There was nothing for me to relate it to.

The doctor continued, 'Unfortunately, there is nothing we can do and patients succumb to the disease in stages. I am afraid you husband is not likely live more than five years.'

Five years! Only five years? I gulped. My eyes narrowed. The doctor was not certain and with the strength John still had, and his lucid episodes when it appeared there was absolutely nothing wrong with him, I doubted if John would succumb to this disease as easily as the doctor thought. But who was I to say?

As soon as I could I dashed to the library. I looked up the disease. My feelings of panic and insecurity needed feeding with information. The more I knew, the more we could fight this dreadful disease.

I read:

'It was named after Arnold Pick who described the condition at the beginning of the twentieth century ... In some families it has a genetic inheritance.' Was this the secret the family held? Or was their secretiveness just their inward-looking nature? Was this something to do with the mystery Uncle Jim? Perhaps this was the disease Uncle Jim had had? I read on: 'Early symptoms are of a change in the personality which often leads to inappropriate or uninhibited behaviour.' John's personality was getting more and more eccentric rather than changing but he was always a gentleman and yet some of the things he was doing and saying were often quite inappropriate.

'Particular areas of the brain degenerate, especially parts of the frontal and temporal lobes.' I always thought when John had a fit that he lost part of his brain. Maybe his fits were a result of this gradual deterioration. Gosh, this was a horrible disease.

'Patient's memory is relatively mildly impaired.' Yes, that was John. He still had a phenomenal memory.

'Early on there may be a loss of judgement, leading to the person appearing rather silly, or putting themselves in dangerous situations without any concern for safety.' Yes, that was John. Lately he was caught quite happily balancing at the top of a ladder or the roof of the shed without any care.

'The person may seem not to care about anything.' Maybe this was why he seemed to be so hard-hearted in our early days? But he really did care for his mother and for me in his own way. He certainly cared when Musta was killed on the road outside our house; we both shared a deep sense of mourning. I was convinced of this. He could care. But did he care about anything now? I wasn't sure.

'Later, problems of speech emerge; carrying out practical tasks becomes more difficult.' Speech definitely wasn't a problem at the moment. The problem was that he wouldn't stop speaking. Even when he worked for the chemical company, they complained of his 'verbal diarrhoea' in his reports.

As for practical tasks, he did seem to be unable to take the same interest in the garden that he had when we first set up house.

'Memory problems seem to develop at a later stage.' That'll be great. I closed the book and sat down on one of the library chairs. I looked around at the people reading quietly, changing their books or sitting at the desks reading newspapers. Why us? Why John? All these people were all right. Life is not fair. I leant over the desk. I tried to think of the future but my mind was swamped with overwhelming darkness.

One Wednesday, when it had been raining constantly and the games I was supposed to supervise had been cancelled, I was allowed the time off and I came home early. I caught the mail. There was an official brown envelope from the Institute of Health. What did Harriet want now? Maybe she was going to help now?

'In spite of your refusal on two separate occasions, the committee has decided to offer respite for John again for one week,' I read. Two other occasions? Oh, John! What had he been doing with the mail? I turned to the letter again. 'He will be collected on the 15th and taken to a home in Suffolk for a short break.' Suffolk? Why Suffolk? I shrugged my shoulders. At least it was somewhere and I knew about it this time. I smiled. He would be away for a whole week.

After he had been there three days, a postcard arrived in the post:

'A game from a friend in the holiday camp:

$2 + 7 + 6 = 15$

$9 + 5 + 1 = 15$

$4 + 3 + 8 = 15$

15 15 15 15'

The following day, there was a message on the phone.

'I'm sorry, Mrs Wilks, your husband has not settled in very well. He will be coming home tomorrow.'

'Now what has he been up to?' I groaned. I phoned the respite centre.

'I'm so sorry, but we have to consider the other patients too,' the nurse's voice was kind. 'He took apart a bicycle owned by one of the staff and hid some of the parts. We're still looking for them.'

On the day he came back another post card came in the post.

'Ernie knew what I did with the bicycle,' John said. 'He asked me, what's the difference between hills and pills? Hills go up, pills go down.'

We resumed our stressful lives together, the girls and I getting on with life as best we could while we tried to cope with John's erratic and aggressive behaviour, trying to remember the occasional moments when he was amusing and trying to ignore or overcome the moments when we hung our heads in embarrassment and shame.

Chapter 37

Then one ordinary school night everything changed.

It was midnight and I was trying to sleep. John was in bed in the next room. His radio was tuned to Radio 4 and was blaring out so loud that the entire neighbourhood could hear it. I had to do something. He had to turn it down. I knew that by this time, if I went and asked him nicely to turn it down, nothing would happen. He was almost impervious to others' needs. The only way I knew how to get him to react to a request was to issue a teacher-type command. I reluctantly dragged myself out of bed. I urgently needed sleep. I went to the open doorway of his room.

In a firm, no-nonsense voice I said, 'You!' He ignored me. 'You!' I shouted, making sure that he knew it was him I was talking to. 'Turn that radio down *now*!'

He stared at me, his eyes wide. He automatically reached out for the switch on the radio and turned it off. He paused. Then his face changed. It contorted into a wild creature, nothing like the man I knew. His chest filled with air and he rose like a tortured bear.

'I'll show you, turn your radio off!' He yelled. He slowly slid his legs from under the bedcovers to the floor. His wild eyes flashed at me. I had never seen him so angry and this anger was focused on me. My heart thumped loudly in my chest. There was no doubt this was John's run-for-cover look, a look that told me I had to get away from him as quickly as possible before he lashed out. This time it was worse than I had ever seen.

Nothing would stop him. This was not the John I had always known. This was an angry madman.

I ran for my room, shut the door quickly and looked around for something to barricade the door with. My heart hammered louder and louder. I grabbed the chair and put it under the door handle. With heavy threatening footsteps he lumbered out of his room, along the landing to my door, his angry voice bellowing 'I'll get you!' I pushed hard against the chair my shoulders aching. My breathing quickened as I pulled back, only my hip firmly against the chair. I stretched one hand away from the barricade to reach for the phone. I stretched hard. I just managed to grip the receiver.

'I'll show you!' The voice outside screamed. He hammered on the door. I put my foot hard against the chair. My fingers shook as I leaned over and dialled the doctor's emergency number.

'Who do you think you are? What are you doing behind your door? I'll stop you, I'll stop you,' he screamed.

'H-hello,' I stuttered, 'it's Mrs Wilks, Witchford, and I need help with John *now*.'

'Who are you phoning?' John's voice paused and he was silent as if suddenly planning his next move. Maybe he was tired? I prayed. Please, God, please make him go to sleep.

'I'll...' The voice trailed off and I heard John's laboured steps go back to his room. I could still hear his voice muttering in muted threatening tones, but at least he was not trying to break down my door. The hammering in my chest eased a little, but I felt vulnerable, very vulnerable. Oh how I hoped the doctor would come soon, very soon. Once John had been given a sedative, he would sleep properly and I would not be under any more threats tonight. At least he wasn't threatening the girls.

I sat on the bed, the chair still firmly jammed against the door and waited for the doorbell.

The ticking of my clock was louder than I had ever heard it before.

Then the doorbell rang. I listened for John. He was silent, too silent. The doorbell rang again. I had to move. I took in a deep breath, pulled the chair back, opened my door slowly and listened. There was no sound. I scuttled as fast as I could past John's room downstairs and opened the front door. I did not dare look into John's room in case it stirred him into chasing me again.

A tall dark figure stood on the doorstep, black bag in his hand.

'Thank you *so* much for coming,' I gasped. 'He has been diagnosed with Pick's disease,' I told the doctor as we walked up the stairs in single file. 'All he needs is sedation.'

'I could do without being dragged out at this hour of the night,' the doctor snapped.

I stood outside the room as the doctor approached John. John was lying in his bed, his eyes still flickering wildly. His silence was sinister.

The doctor spoke to him. John replied, adding in a spine-chilling tone, 'I'll stop her using the phone.'

There was only one way I could think of stopping me using the phone and I was certain that if he succeeded I would not remain alive that night. One blow from John, who had never really understood his strength, and I would be dead; there was no doubt about that in my mind.

The doctor stood up. I stared at him open-mouthed. He came out of the room.

'Your husband does not want to be sedated and I will not sedate him against his will.' I could hardly believe my ears.

'I – I'm so frightened that if you leave this house, I-I will leave too,' I stuttered.

'I'll get the police,' the doctor muttered and walked down the stairs. I followed him. He opened the door and let himself out. I clutched the keys and watched the doctor's back as he climbed into his car and sped off. Standing in my pyjamas and dressing gown on our front doorstep I could not get myself to return to the house. It was too dangerous. I went into the garage and sat in the car. No, this was not safe enough. I could imagine John rushing downstairs and round to the car to yank my door open.

I drove out of the garage. John could still easily storm downstairs and try to fling open the car door. I locked the car doors. I was still not safe. With his super strength he could easily smash the window open. I looked back at the house. If I were a proper mother I would stay in the house to protect the children. But it was not the children he was determined to 'stop'. It was me. If I removed the focus of his anger, maybe things would quieten down. I drove the car to the edge of the driveway. It would only take a few seconds for John to rush out and attack the car.

I drove across the road and parked within sight of the house. I kept the keys in the ignition. If I saw John rush out of the house I could probably drive away in time. My instinct was to drive away right now, as far away as possible until I felt safe. But I could not do this. I had to be near in case he tried to hit the girls. However, I was sure it was only me that he had in mind to attack, but could I be sure? I was ashamed of my cowardice. I should be in the house ready to protect the girls. I reasoned that as long as I stayed within sight of the two upstairs rooms I would be able to go back in and rescue them if I had to. I compromised. I decided that if I saw either of the girls' lights go on, no matter how afraid I felt, I had to go back inside and deal with him. Would I be able to do this? I would be no match for John's strength. I tried to make myself comfortable in the seat of the car and stared at the girls' windows. They remained in darkness. In spite of my fear, my eyes drooped. I had a fitful night's sleep.

I awoke, cold and uncomfortable, the fear still present. I looked up at the girls' windows on the second floor. There were no lights on. The street was empty. I tentatively opened the car door. There was no reaction. The front door of the house was firmly closed. Would John be standing behind the door still determined to attack? The last time I saw him he was in bed. Perhaps he had stayed in bed and would still be asleep. I really hoped so.

Glancing to the right and left I walked quickly across the road. There were no other cars and none of the neighbours was out yet. I put the key into the door and carefully opened it. The house was silent. I got the breakfasts ready as quietly as I could. No one came downstairs. I was getting braver by the minute. Finally, I crept up the stairs and peeked around John's door. He was in bed. Thank goodness! I could not be absolutely sure he was sound asleep but he did not respond as I peeked in. I withdrew quickly and woke the girls.

'Shh, we have to be very quiet. Your dad is not well. Are you all right?'

A bleary-eyed face tried to focus on me.

'Yes, I'm okay. Dad threw the cat at me last night,' said Penny drowsily.

'Sorry.' I didn't go into what had happened the previous night. The girls had probably heard it for themselves. They must have been cowering in their beds, poor things. I was relieved that the worst John did was get annoyed enough to pick up the poor animal and throw it on one of the girl's beds. I must have been right — it was me, and only me he was ready to attack.

The girls and I managed to get dressed without John stirring. We went downstairs, ate our breakfasts as quietly as we could and got ready for school, albeit more hurriedly than usual. I put John's breakfast on a tray and went upstairs. I stood at the entrance of the room, ready to run if I needed. John lay in bed. He was still but breathing. I put his breakfast tray on the floor at the entrance to the room.

'John!' I called. He stirred and mumbled. He was still not happy.

'I've left your breakfast here in the doorway. Can you go to Dinah's?'

I did not wait for a reply. I shepherded the girls outside and to the car and we drove off to school as quickly as we could. We were early for school that day, for a change.

I stayed at school as long as possible, avoiding the prospect of seeing John again. As we drove home I prayed that John would not be there. What would I do if he were? I decided that we would not go into the house if he were there. We would have to arrive on a friend's doorstep. Oh, how I hoped John had gone to Dinah's.

The house was empty. What a relief. I went into 'automatic' mode. I was determined that I would provide a decent home for the girls no matter what. I started doing the chores. We would go through the usual routine as if we were not affected by what had happened. While I brought in the washing from the line, I folded it and wondered what was going to happen next. I could not risk having John home again. What was going to happen to him? Dinah could not have him staying with her forever.

I took the laundry upstairs and put it in the airing cupboard or in the ironing pile. I went downstairs and started preparing dinner for us. The phone rang. It was Dinah.

'I thought you ought to know, they've taken John into hospital. He didn't want to go; the doctors had to section him.'

Chapter 38

I felt numb. I expected to feel a great sense of relief. Yes, I was relieved and felt more secure, but I was also swept with a feeling a great sadness. My John, the man who brought sparkle and excitement into our lives, was reduced to an angry and confused patient in a hospital. It was so sad. It was so unfair. He had never wished to harm anyone. He was the one who always wanted to be involved in helping others. He did not deserve this.

I shook off these feelings. Feeling sorry for oneself never achieved anything. Besides, I had to be both father and mother to the children now. I busied myself with the household chores and with arranging visits to see John in the hospital.

I avoided going at first. Fortunately I had the excuse that the doctors had asked us to leave him there for a bit before we saw him but I knew that when the time came when we could visit, I was still stalling. I did not want to see him in this state and I still felt afraid that he might hurt me. I still felt frightened that he would escape the ward and walk home. He certainly had the strength, stamina and determination to do this. Fifty or so miles would be nothing to him if he were determined enough.

One day, soon after John had been taken to hospital, the phone rang.

'Did you know,' the nurse's voice sounded agitated, 'it took six of us to hold him down? It usually only takes two!'

'I believe you,' I replied. What else could I say? Why did she call? Was she asking *me* for sympathy? Well, she certainly had my sympathy but how could I help? I was not a trained nurse. In fact if you were looking for someone with nursing skills, you were looking at the wrong person. I have always been a coward where injury and nursing are concerned. Nevertheless, I felt vindicated. John was in hospital for good reason. If it took six of them to hold him down, how on earth was I supposed to cope on my own at home?

'When will Daddy be coming home?' Emma asked as we were on our way to visit him.

'I don't know' I said, changing gear. I could see Emma lean back in her seat, her mouth down, her arms folded close to her body.

'You know it is not Daddy that has been the trouble, it is his illness. It is his illness that has made the doctors put Daddy in hospital. If your daddy were all right he would still be with us. It's his illness that we are fighting.'

When we arrived John stood next to one of the walls of the communal areas. The girls stuck close to me as other patients wandered aimlessly around the stark room, living in their own confused worlds. John was still in a highly agitated state. He looked particularly worried about something.

'Is there something troubling you?' I asked.

'They won't let me show them how I can dress myself.'

'That —' I did not have time to finish my sentence. Two members of staff swiftly ran to John, standing either side of him.

'Er, what's up?' I asked the staff member on the right.

'Oh, when John wants to show that he can dress himself, he insists on hitting the fire alarm. We've had the fire brigade out twice already.'

Good old John, I thought, keep them busy.

The following visit he confidentially informed me that the Duke of Edinburgh was standing in front of him. I stopped myself from laughing at him, smiled and tried to sound sympathetic. At least I knew he was in the right place.

One Wednesday, after a rather arduous day of extra rehearsals for a school concert coming up, we arrive home to a phone message.

'It's the staff nurse here.' The voice was calm and matter-of-fact. 'We found John with his face bruised. He has had a massive fit and banged his face on the radiator next to his bed. He is in Ward Six at the hospital.'

The following day the children went to Babs and I went to the hospital alone. I found his ward on the third floor. There was no one about. The central desk to the ward was unattended and each adjoining room contained people who were unconscious like John. John lay inert on the bed a catheter inserted. He was still breathing.

I looked around the ward. Still nobody came. It would be no good getting cross; there was probably a staff shortage as usual. Impatient, I decided to do something about the situation. I leaned over the desk and picked up the phone.

'Hello?' I said in a friendly cheeky voice.

'Who is that?' the official voice asked.

'Well, I'm just a visitor to Ward Six and there is nobody, absolutely nobody at the desk.'

'But there must be!'

'Nope, and I can see all these confidential papers about the patients on the desk.'

'Look, someone *must* be there.'

'Nope, nobody yet and there are a lot of patients in the ward. They all look terribly ill.'

The tone of the speaker changed. 'Well,' he said in a patronizing tone, 'I think you have been on the phone long enough now. Put the phone down and I will see what I can do.' I laughed. He obviously though I was a psychiatric patient playing mischief.

A tiny nurse eventually scuttled past to the end room. Well, there was one member of staff here at least.

I put a framed photo of the girls and I next to John's bed, patted his inert arm and went home.

At the weekend the three of us visited him. The framed photo was in place but the picture of me had been taken out and left on the table. John was still inert in the bed. How did he do that? It was very unlikely any of the staff had time or inclination to do such a strange thing. There was no accounting for what John could do while still in a fit.

Emma and I went on the third visit. Penny had to play for the school hockey team and was not ready to see her dad in that state yet.

Emma and I walked to the ward. We looked at his bed. It was empty, with the mattress rolled up.

'Well, Emma,' I tried to sound cheerful, 'he's either dead or they've moved him.'

'Mum!' Emma looked up at me, alarmed.

'Don't worry, I'm sure they've moved him but they've forgotten to tell us.'

The little nurse scurried towards us. I put a hand out mid-flight and asked 'Where is John Wilks?'

'Oh, they've moved him.'

'Could you tell me to which ward, please?'

'No, sorry. I'll just see to this patient and then I'll look it up.'

Emma and I waited until we were told John's new ward and we made our way there.

He looked much better. He was sitting on the edge of his bed his hands firmly by his side looking like a schoolboy who had just been caught out.

'What's up? Have you been a naughty boy?' I teased.

'I wanted to go for a walk,' he said.

'That seems a reasonable request. Perhaps one of the staff could have accompanied you. Where did you want to go?'

He pointed to the window. Ah, that explains their reticence. He had wanted to go out of the window and it seemed reasonable enough for the staff to prevent him, especially considering we were three floors above the ground!

On the following visit to the ward, John started to talk about a carrot.

'Look', he said, 'there's a big carrot in the corridor.' I looked. There was no carrot. I had remembered the doctors seemed especially interested in John's realistic dreams. They seemed to be closely connected with his fits. I thought I should warn the staff.

A young staff member was busying herself at the desk.

'I think I ought to report that John is having hallucinations. He is seeing a carrot in the corridor.'

'Oh, that's not having hallucinations,' she snapped pompously. 'That's inappropriate behaviour.'

I stared hard at her. She did not blink. I thought of responding with 'Go on then, show me the carrot,' but thought better of it. It crossed my mind that it was sometimes difficult to tell who ought to be looking after whom in this crazy ward.

John was eventually returned to the mental hospital.

After one of our regular visits, the doctor sat at his desk, holding his glasses.

'John will be all right with us. We will see to him. You have no need to worry. He needs a stable environment, which we can provide. He will be with us indefinitely, probably for the rest of his life. You know,' he confided, 'looking at the file it seems your doctors in Ely had been thinking of sectioning him at least two weeks before they did. It must have been very difficult for you.'

I sat absolutely still. Then without warning I suddenly burst into tears. The doctor stayed seated, his calm figure waiting patiently until the last of my sobs. The clock on the wall ticked loudly. I pulled out a handkerchief and wiped away my tears. As I composed myself, another feeling crept over me. Mixed with a terrible sadness was a feeling of tremendous relief. I swallowed. I thought guiltily, if I were a really loyal and sympathetic wife I should fight to have him home. Images of that terrible night when he was determined to attack me flashed in my mind. No, he was in the right place.

The following week I picked up the post. It was such a relief to know that I would receive all the letters delivered to our address. One of the letters was a familiar brown envelope from the Institute of Health. It was probably a letter from Harriet Bendall confirming what the doctor had said. But it wasn't. Open mouthed I read the contents.

'The mental hospital has finished with his assessment so he needs to be moved. We are sorry that you refuse to come to our meetings, so we are writing to you as you requested to tell you that we are moving him to a mental institution in Norfolk.'

I sat down. Why so far away? It would take hours to drive there to see him.

The doorbell rang.

'Hi,' Babs' cheerful face grinned. 'I was just passing and brought a thermos of coffee and some cakes. Got five minutes?'

'Oh, Babs,' I cried, 'I'm so pleased to see you. Come in.' I listened to the girls who were talking animatedly upstairs but no argument had developed yet.

Babs poured me a cup of coffee and handed it to me. I was still clutching the letter.

'Here,' I said, holding the letter out to Babs. 'What do you make of this?'

'Oh, that would be Heil Harriets.' She grimaced. 'They don't want to pay for John so they are shunting him to a new county.'

'But the doctor said he should have a stable environment. He should stay where he is.'

'That would be right, but you don't think Harriet would let a little thing like that worry her, do you?' Babs sipped her own coffee. 'The doctors are up in arms, but they are being ignored.'

The day John was moved was sunny. I arrived at the hospital ready to accompany him so that he felt more secure. He was subdued for the whole journey. We were approaching the seafront.

'Could we let John have a walk by the sea?' I asked the driver.

'Of course we can.' The driver stopped the car.

'Come on, John,' I touched John's hand, 'let's go for a walk on the beach.' My heart was heavy. This would probably be the last time John would see the sea, something he loved and that meant so much to him. I thought of the holidays he had enjoyed so much at Butlin's when the girls were much younger and when he managed to be free from his fits.

'No,' John said firmly, but without anger.

'The nurse and I will be with you. You'll be all right,' I said, looking into his troubled face.

He hung his head, his cheeks went white. 'No,' he said, 'no.' He was a broken man.

The mental hospital was up a steep hill. The car pulled into the car park and the nurse, John and I entered the hospital. On the right was a sitting area. A woman was sitting directly opposite us and she reminded me of someone — his mother! She sat primly on the edge of her seat, her eagle eyes defying anyone to come near her. Her face must have been graceful and charming once, but now it was pinched and angry.

'Come in, John' the nurse greeting us said.

John walked towards the woman. 'Waiting for Christmas, are you?' John said, sitting next to her.

'Don't be silly. What do you think you're doing here? Get out of that chair.' I gasped at the electrical sparks that were flying between them. I could not understand how this could be a better place for him, but I had no say. This was to be John's home and there was nothing I could do about it. How was I going to get the time to bring the girls to see him here? I decided, whatever we had to do, we must visit John in this alarming atmosphere.

Chapter 39

A few days later there was a message on the phone.

I recognized Harriet's voice immediately. 'The institution in Norfolk has been found wanting. John is being moved into a ward in a Cambridge hospital tomorrow.' I grimaced. Another move for him — what were they doing?

I wrote yet another letter of complaint. It was ignored.

After he had settled into the ward, another letter arrived. This time he was going to be moved out because they were closing the ward. This happened two more times.

'There won't be any more wards left at this rate,' I laughed to Babs, my laughter tinged with hysteria.

'I think you might be right,' she said seriously. This was the first time I had seen Babs worried.

The following Saturday the phone rang.

'Is that Mrs Wilks?' a smooth female voice asked hesitantly.

'Yes,' I said, equally hesitantly.

'It's Mrs Davidson here.'

'Yes?' I was trying to remember who she was.

'I have recently been appointed in charge of John's ward. I don't know what to do. The ward is being closed down and he is the last patient left.'

I remained silent. What could I do?

'I just thought you ought to know. We'll let you know what happens.'

Now I was angry. What were they playing at? John needed that ward; he needed to have stability and a regular pattern to his life. How dare they shunt him from place to place like a piece of furniture? They will just have to find somewhere for him.

Harriet's cold tones echoed from the answer machine two days later.

'Your husband is in a private home in Norton.'

Two days later Harriet's letter arrived demanding payment for John's care.

'Surely the Health Institution is responsible for him?' I said to Babs over coffee the next day. They were the ones that insisted on this change. He had worked all his life as long as he could and paid his way. He was entitled to free health care, surely?

'Yes, I think you're right,' Babs replied. 'There was a court case about this which a patient called Pamela Coughlin won. John is much worse than she was but in spite of that Harriet and her cronies are devising more ways of getting the patients' families to cough up.' She grimaced. 'Some people are being made to sell their homes.'

I suddenly felt cold. What would we do if we were turned out of our home? This would *not* happen. Every weekend I pored over the paperwork, making sure John paid expenses the institution was entitled to, and replying to every letter I received making demands with a query.

The most recent letter I received said, 'If you don't complete this document correctly and immediately, you will be liable to pay all of the institution's fees, some £600 a week.'

'Six hundred pounds a week?' I shrieked at Babs. 'We don't have that kind of money! What can I do?'

'You stick to your guns, girl.' Babs patted my hand. 'Keep appealing. Maybe you should go to one of the meetings.'

'No, I don't think that would be a good idea. At least I'll have evidence if I keep insisting on everything being in writing.'

'Would you like me to go to a meeting as your representative?'

'Oh, would you Babs? That would be wonderful. Maybe they will listen to you.'

At the end of the week, another brown envelope came. 'With regard to the protection of client John Wilks.'

"Client," I muttered to myself, why ever call him a "client"? He's a patient, a human being. And what do they mean by "protection"? They're hardly protecting him the way they have been treating him and the way they're harassing his family.

I read on. 'The next meeting will be held on Monday 20th of this month. You and your representative are invited to attend. In the meantime you are informed that on no account are your husband's funds to be used for anything for his family, he is not permitted to contribute to gifts of any kind...' the list went on. I could hardly believe it. Who was Harriet to say what John could or could not do? She was never married to the man, I was. Besides, not only was I vulnerable as the wife of someone terminally ill, I was being harassed — where was the compassion and care this so-called caring society was supposed to show?

I picked up the telephone.

'Hello,' Babs said quickly.

'It's Sally. You know you offered to go to a meeting for me...?'

I paced up and down in the sitting room. The girls were upstairs supposedly doing their homework. As long as they were quiet, I did not interfere. I had more to worry about. The doorbell finally rang. I rushed to the door and flung it open. Babs stepped quickly inside.

'Well,' she said taking a deep breath as she sat on the sofa. 'Talk about a lynching. Now I know why you wouldn't attend meetings.'

I perched on the edge of the chair. 'Why? What happened?'

'Heil Harriet was in fine form. John was hardly mentioned. They wanted to know all about you and what you have done with his money, you wicked girl you.' She laughed. I grimaced.

'They've never asked me directly for a financial statement on John's money. Why all this fuss now?'

'I told them that John was perfectly entitled to free care, but they didn't want to know. Then they said they were getting the police onto you.'

'The police? But what have I done?'

'I think it was all bluff, but I would be on the safe side if I were you.'

'Oh, Babs.' My shoulders tensed and my eyes watered. 'What if they demand everything they've paid already towards John's care? It would come to thousands of pounds, which I simply do not have. I'm only just managing to cover the mortgage as it is and look after the girls.'

'Look,' Babs came across to me. 'You and I know you've done nothing wrong. Just hang in there. Things will sort themselves out and if it comes to the worst, we can bail you out. Pots of money, that's what we've got, but don't tell anyone.' Her dark eyes twinkled, 'We would have to negotiate the interest, of course.'

'Oh thanks, Babs,' I blubbered.

I walked on a tightrope for months. Everything I did I tried to see through Heil Harriet's eyes. I could not afford a single mistake. The girls' and my home was at risk.

'What's the matter, Mum?' Penny asked over dinner one evening. 'You look pale.'

'It's all right, Penny,' I said, 'we're going through a difficult time with your father, but it will all work out in the end.' I gulped. I did not really believe what I had said, but I had to keep up appearances for the girls. They had enough on their plates with having to suffer the indignity of the knowledge that their father had gone mad and was now incapacitated in a home. They were bound to have been taunted with this knowledge by their unkind classmates.

The phone rang. I slowly picked up the receiver, praying it was not more bad news.

'Seen tonight's paper?' Babs spluttered.

'No, once John left I cancelled the nightly paper. I have no time to read it.'

'Stay there!' she laughed. 'I'll bring it over.'

'Who was that?' Emma asked.

'Just Babs. She's coming over.'

'Can we watch TV?' Penny asked.

'Yes, you can watch TV. We'll go into the dining room.'

I unloaded the dishwasher and put away the clean dishes. I wiped down the kitchen sink, something I had not done for ages. I usually left it to the cleaning lady whose sole job was to keep the house from becoming a health risk. I tidied the sitting room, removing everything off the floor around the girls, who were glued to the TV. I worked like an obsessive housewife until the doorbell finally rang. I rushed to the door.

'Here!' Babs grinned. 'Read the headlines.'

I steadied the paper that she had thrust into my hands. 'Head of Institute of Health charged with theft.'

'Come in, come in,' I said, clutching the paper and trying to read as we moved to the dining room. We sat down. I looked at the first sentence 'Harriet Bendall ...' Mouth open I stared at Babs. 'You mean Heil Harriet has been caught stealing?'

'Yes. She was extricating money from families like yours and putting it into her own bank account.'

'Wow! No more horrible letters from Harriet Bendall!' I hugged Babs. 'I'm free!'

'Of course you are, you idiot, and now maybe they'll make people like her follow a Code of Practice like other large institutions have to.'

'Maybe.' I sat down. A huge black cloud that had been clinging to my shoulders since John had first been sectioned suddenly disappeared. In one single moment, I was released. I laughed.

The figure in the bed beside me turned towards me, coughed and smiled. Had John sensed the joy that I remembered feeling on that wonderful day?

I looked at him and his smile broadened further. His eyes twinkled with love. There was no aggression this time. He did not grab my hand or bang on the side of the bed. He let me put my hand on his and for one long moment we looked at each other.

I could have sworn that in this single moment he fully understood my feelings and I knew that whatever there existed between us when we first married was here with us in this care home room now, wrapping itself round us like a huge warm cloak. We were together, husband and wife. Whatever the future held, nothing would be able to detract from the feelings we had for each other in this brief moment.

END

Postscript

Since Pamela Coughlan won her case against the British government in 1999, it has been established that when the primary need for a patient is healthcare and they need accommodation in a nursing home, the NHS is responsible for the full cost. Pamela Coughlin's condition was less severe than John's. But even though John qualified for Continuing Care, the government representatives dealing with his case did not and could not be persuaded to apply the law.

With the help of solicitor Henry Anstey of HC Solicitors in Peterborough, Rosemary was able to appeal against John's assessment. He was finally awarded continuing care costs and the government body was instructed to pay the solicitor's fees. s

For more information, contact:

www.hcsolicitors.co.uk